"In *Not Wanting a Thing to be the Thing*, Mitzi J. Smith shares her deeply personal journey as a stroke survivor, weaving together the intersection of health disparities, trauma, faith, and resilience within the Black community. Written from her perspective as a Black woman, biblical scholar, and womanist writer, this creative memoir explores the profound impact of stroke on the body, mind, and soul. Smith's story is a necessary act of survival, offering a raw, poignant reflection on healing, survival, and the fight for justice."

—DONALD E. QUIST
Author of *To Those Bounded*

"Smith's stroke memoir recounts her experience of the 'civil war' within her body and her subsequent recovery. With unflinching honesty and vulnerability, Smith provides a bold voice for the many voiceless patients from whom we all must learn. This moving and inspiring memoir should be assigned reading for all healthcare professionals and student clinicians."

—AMY BECKLENBERG
Clinical Associate Professor, Marcella Niehoff School of Nursing,
Loyola University Chicago

"In this remarkable stroke memoir, Dr. Mitzi Smith reflects on her struggle and survival through the lenses of intergenerational history, biblical texts, and medical realities. The result is a piercing and poignant fight story, an act of vulnerability and courage, and a generous sharing of hard-earned wisdom that will inspire and empower anyone who faces life-changing trauma."

—CHRISTINE ROY YODER
Senior Vice President, Columbia Theological Seminary

"As a sixty-something black woman who has recently had to accept the fact that there are some ailments that now require medication, I hungrily attached myself to Mitzi's story in a way that surprised me, in a way that brought tears to my eyes. I had secretly wondered whether she would write about her 'thing' that she didn't want to be a thing and oh did she ever. Mitzi is a brilliant thinker and riveting writer, and so all her writings have left a part of me forever changed—but this book is personal. In her own words, this is her 'fight story.' A story indeed about the 'civil war' that erupted in her body. Mitzi has never been one to hold back, but this level of transparency invites every woman to the emergency room where their sacred scars can find a community of hearers. It's been said that every winner has scars. Thank you, Mitzi, for sharing yours with us and challenging us to fess up and deal with our things that we didn't want to be a thing."

—GENETTA Y. HATCHER
Pastor, The Room Church, Roseville, Michigan

"Mitzi Smith's transparency is a great gift in this riveting, must-read memoir. Her discussion of 'the wars that broke out in my body' weaves a testimonial of vulnerability with threads of faith-filled resiliency and loving memories of her mother. Identifying as an '"intergenerational creative and fighter,' Smith's poignant message of humble gratitude for each milestone also boldly unveils the inconsistencies of healthcare systems. This memoir inspires us to navigate life's dance of uncertainty with hope."

—VALERIE MILES-TRIBBLE
Professor of Ministerial Leadership and Practical Theology, Graduate Theological Union, Berkeley School of Theology

"Shaped by experiential knowing that is informed by a keen awareness of complex systems that disproportionately affect the lives of Black women, *Not Wanting a Thing to Be the Thing* is a fight story—a revolutionary act born out of a desire to live and thrive. The author's transparency, vulnerability, and resiliency serve as a warning to Black women, and those who love them, to be attentive to and responsive to one's body."

—ANGELA D. SIMS
President, Colgate Rochester Crozer Divinity School

# Not Wanting *a* Thing to Be *the* Thing

# Not Wanting *a* Thing to Be *the* Thing

An African American Woman
Biblical Scholar's Stroke Memoir

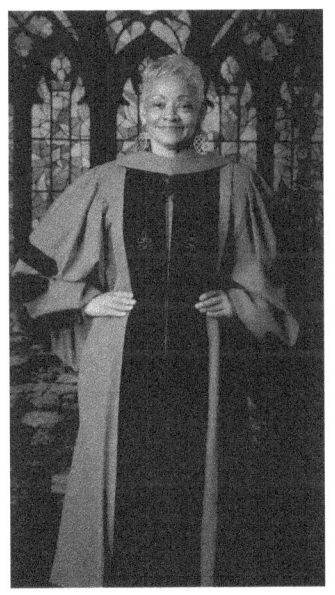

MITZI J. SMITH

*Foreword by J. Alfred Smith Sr.*

CASCADE *Books* • Eugene, Oregon

NOT WANTING A THING TO BE THE THING
An African American Woman Biblical Scholar's Stroke Memoir

Copyright © 2025 Mitzi J. Smith. All rights reserved. Except for brief quotations in critical publications or reviews, no part of this book may be reproduced in any manner without prior written permission from the publisher. Write: Permissions, Wipf and Stock Publishers, 199 W. 8th Ave., Suite 3, Eugene, OR 97401.

Cascade Books
An Imprint of Wipf and Stock Publishers
199 W. 8th Ave., Suite 3
Eugene, OR 97401

www.wipfandstock.com

PAPERBACK ISBN: 979-8-3852-3641-1
HARDCOVER ISBN: 979-8-3852-3642-8
EBOOK ISBN: 979-8-3852-3643-5

*Cataloguing-in-Publication data:*

Names: Smith, Mitzi J., author. | Smith, J. Alfred, Sr., foreword.

Title: Not wanting a thing to be the thing : an African American woman biblical scholar's stroke memoir / Mitzi J. Smith, author; foreword by J. Alfred Smith Sr.

Description: Eugene, OR: Cascade Books, 2025 | Includes bibliographical references.

Identifiers: ISBN 979-8-3852-3641-1 (paperback) | ISBN 979-8-3852-3642-8 (hardcover) | ISBN 979-8-3852-3643-5 (ebook)

Subjects: LCSH: Mitzi J. Smith, 1957– —Health. | Cerebrovascular disease—Patient—United States—Biography. | Bible—Hermeneutics. | Minorities—Medical care—United States.

Classification: RC388.5 S65 2025 (paperback) | RC388.5 (ebook)

VERSION NUMBER 060925

# Contents

*List of Illustrations* | ix
*Foreword* | xi
*Acknowledgments* | xiii
*Introduction—A Necessary Act: A Black Woman's Stroke Memoir* | xv

**Part 1—Not Wanting *a* Thing to Be *the* Thing
    Doesn't Make It Something Else**

1   I *Am* My Mother; I *Am Not* My Mother | 3
2   Civil War | 5
3   Terror | 7
4   Stroke Symptoms in Women | 10
5   It Might Be a Stroke | 12
6   Urgent Care | 14
7   Showing Up | 17
8   The ER: I Can't Write My Name | 21
9   Quadruple Risk | 26
10  They Don't Serve Food in the ICU | 28
11  Fight | 30
12  My Mother Was a Nurse; I Wanted to Be Like Her | 32
13  Not On My Watch | 35
14  From ICU to a Bed in EH | 37

**Part 2—Recovery Begins: Emory Hospital**

15  Somebody Prayed for Me | 41
16  Blood, Sodium, and Water | 44

17  Can't Feed Myself! | 46
18  Day Two: Angels | 47
19  God Didn't Cause Me to Have a Stroke | 50
20  Day Three: Retaliation | 52
21  Left Alone | 54
22  Another Angel | 56
23  Physical Therapy Begins | 58
24  Outside World | 60
25  Ready for Rehab | 62

**Part 3—Fighting My Way Back: Emory Rehabilitation Hospital**
26  Arrival | 65
27  Dr. Justin and the Quiz | 67
28  (Dis)Respect, Patient Preference, and Gender | 68
29  Dr. Milton and Still Me | 70
30  Rhythm and Rhyme of Therapy | 73
31  Noise | 74
32  A Shelterless Black Woman Cleans My Room | 77
33  Occupational Therapy | 79
34  Speech Therapy | 82
35  Physical Therapy and Walking | 85
36  Meal Plan | 88
37  Lucky | 90
38  Doctor in the House? | 94
39  Paul and Georgia | 97
40  Tears | 101
41  Visitors | 104
42  Two Days Before I'm Discharged: I Still Need Help! | 107
43  Discharge from ERH | 111

**Part 4—Home and Nineteen Months Later**
44  My Help Cometh From Sina! | 117
45  Meal Train, DoorDash, and Chicken Soup | 120
46  "Is this the hardest thing you've ever done?" | 122

47  Outpatient Therapy | 123
48  Back in the Classroom | 128
49  Palimpsest | 130
50  Facebook Updates: Stroke Recovery Progress | 132
51  Kidney Disease?! | 139
52  Fragments | 142
53  Epilogue | 149

*Appendix—Reproductive Justice, Medical Apartheid, and the Gospel of Matthew* | 153

*Bibliography* | 169

# List of Illustrations

Figure 01: Mitzi Jane Smith, twenty months post-stroke | iii

Figure 02: Flora Smith when she graduated from high school | 34

Figure 03: Me and my mother, Flora Ophelia Carson Smith | xx

Figure 04: Mommy in her wheelchair with my oldest niece Misty Smith as a young girl | 34

Figure 05: My mother Flora's self-portrait | xx

Figure 06: Me, Sina, and Napria (my great Niece) in the forefront | 127

Figure 07: My mother's grandparents, (Daddy) George and Flora Jane Carson | 34

Figure 08: Me and Mommy | xx

Figure 09: Me at Harvard University as a PhD student studying religion | 96

Figure 10: Me graduating from Harvard with my PhD—Mommy was too ill to travel | 96

Figure 11: Mitzi twenty months post-stroke | 152

Figure 12: Mitzi and younger sister Lenora | 127

# Foreword

No need to ask, "Can I get a witness?" Your spiritual elder brother is a witness! Smith's *Not Wanting a Thing to Be the Thing: An African American Woman Biblical Scholar's Stroke Memoir* is unique and timely. Eleven years ago, in the busy month of September, my overfull schedule abruptly stopped. I had taught my evening preaching class at the American Baptist Seminary of the West (now Berkeley School of Theology), anticipated flying to Los Angeles to speak at the annual meeting of the American Baptist Churches of the Pacific Northwest, and was prepared to preach at the Black Pastors Conference that same week. I never made it to the Oakland Airport to fly to the city of the angels. Early that morning my wife, Bernestine Smith, drove me to the emergency room of Kaiser Hospital in Antioch, California, where doctors discovered that I had an ischemic stroke that paralyzed my left side and left me with mild slurring of my speech. This traumatic experience well qualifies me to be a witness to the efficacy of Dr. Mitzi Smith's stroke memoir.

My own experience parallels many of her stories. Although Smith shares from her respected perspective as a womanist scholar, men can profit much from reading her story as I have done. In fact, her story is priority reading for all ages, since people suffer strokes at any age. When Amy Jones, my oldest daughter, brought to my bedside reading material from persons who were sharing their success, not a single author wrote from the social location and cultural context of the Black experience. And as an academic, Smith shares her story with wit, humor, and warmth, like Jesus whom the common people heard.

When I was active as a pastor, I faced situations where stroke patients lacked the will to cooperate with both physical and occupational therapists to improve. Remembering such understandably defeating feelings and reflecting on how both Mitzi and I cultivate the desire, the self-confidence, resilience, and rest for step-by-step improvement, I am hopeful that her stroke memoir will encourage both patients and their families. Not everyone in stroke recovery is fortunate to have the caregiving support of a faithful compassionate caregiver and advocate. For eleven years, my wife and partner has continued to be an advocate for me with the medical system, and she gently coaches me to continue my daily post-stroke exercises.

I am a witness that my sister Mitzi's *Not Wanting* a *Thing to Be* the *Thing* is an act of social justice and mercy; it will mitigate some health disparities, expose misinformation, and highlight missed information so prevalent in our communities. Her memoir as an act of love is empowerment. She believes that knowledge is power and that power is for all or for none. Some writing by academics obscures the truth with abstract writing styles that affirm the power of the status quo. Whereas, I am a witness that Mitzi utilizes her freedom to help liberate those who may feel traditionally powerless. This womanist perspective will inform and inspire readers. The words of Professor Emerita Marcia Riggs' book title best describes the intentionality of this memoir: *Awake, Arise, and Act*!

Rev. Dr. J. Alfred Smith Sr.<br>
Pastor emeritus, Allen Temple Baptist Church, Oakland, CA<br>
Emeritus professor, Berkeley School of Religion

# Acknowledgments

I AM THANKFUL TO Dr. Lynne Westfield, director of the Wabash Center for Teaching Religion and Theology, for her visionary leadership and the opportunity to attend a week-long creative roundtable at the Serenbe Inn in Georgia in July 2024. Dr. Don Quist and Sophfronia Scott (author of *Wild Beautiful and Free*) served as co-leaders of the roundtable. Quist is a creative writing professor, author of *To Those Bounded* and other books, and the educational design director at Wabash. Their leadership and the camaraderie of peers inspired and equipped me to write this stroke memoir. I learned from Quist and Scott's instruction and conversations, the daily writing exercises, and the time and space allotted us to write and revise, of which I took full advantage. I also greatly benefited from the feedback from and dialogue with my peers in the large group meetings and with Drs. DeAnna Daniels, Valerie Miles-Tribble, and Sarah Farmer as we huddled together.

Thank you, Dr. Renita Weems for your thoughtful feedback after reading a penultimate copy of the manuscript. For the first time in my career, I secured a professional proofreader, Dr. Caroline Blyth. I'm grateful for Caroline's meticulous expertise. However, I take full responsibility for any errors or omissions in the finished project. I'm grateful to Columbia Theological Seminary (CTS) for additional faculty development funds that allowed me to pay for Caroline's services, and for study leave that gave me time to do this and other work.

My CTS colleagues, friends, and students rallied to pray for me and to provide delicious meals through a meal train and gift cards during the earliest two to three weeks of my recovery at home. I'm eternally grateful. Every act of kindness is a healing balm. I am thankful for former students and colleagues who know me from Ashland Theological Seminary's Detroit Center (now closed), where I taught for the first thirteen years of my academic career. Thank you for your tremendous gift, Minister Kizzie Kelly, Pastor Isaiah Pettway, Dr. Eric Williams, Capuccine Dickerson, Doris Ryans, Pastor Harold Cadwell, Cheryl Coleman-Brown, Dr. Franklin Vaughn, Dr. Jacqueline Nelson, Lester Thomas, Lekina Bell, Aaron Moore, MarShondra Lawrence, Sheyonna Watson, LaRon Moore, Minister Al McCann, Pastor Kellen Brooks, Pastor Roslyn Bouier, and others. You remain special to me. I am grateful to Drs. Renee Harrison, Genetta Hatcher, Angela Sims, Abby Myers, Cheryl Ward, Valerie Miles-Tribble, Candida Moss, and so many others for your gifts and constant prayers. I am grateful to Dr. Ralph Watkins, my CTS colleague and a friend, also known as "the scholar with a camera," and his wife Vanessa's constant prayers. Ralph took the amazing photographs of me enhancing this memoir.

Thank you, my friend, Rev. Dr. J. Alfred Smith Sr., pastor emeritus of Allen Temple Baptist Church in Oakland, California. He is also a stroke survivor. Smith is my elder brother. Like my biological brother Fred, he read my books and would let me know that he had. During my illness and recovery, he called to encourage me, pray for me, check on me, share his wisdom, and graciously agreed to write the foreword for my memoir. Smith advised early on, "Don't let anyone interfere with your rest." I have not.

Finally, I am grateful for all my friends, on and off social media, who have prayed and continue to pray for my recovery. I love you all!

Introduction

# A Necessary Act
## A Black Woman's Stroke Memoir

*A writer's life and work are not a gift to [humankind]; they are its necessity.—*
*Toni Morrison, The Source of Self-Regard*

It was not until I suffered a stroke that I became aware of the extensive impact of stroke on Black communities and Americans in general. I didn't realize how many people that I know personally, apart from family members, had suffered a stroke. They are people with whom I grew up, sat next to in church, and with whom I attended high school or college. They are long-time social media friends and followers, colleagues that I've known for years but with whom I lost touch, and relatives of colleagues. Every Black person knows too many people who have suffered a stroke and survived or died. I didn't know how prevalent and disproportionately deadly stroke is for Black women and men.

When family, friends, colleagues, and social media followers learn that I've suffered a stroke, most are surprised. "Not Mitzi," they say in disbelief. Many know that I walk, lift free weights, and do regular push-ups and other weight-bearing exercises at home. They know that I belong to a gym, pay for a personal trainer from time to time, don't eat pork or red meat, don't smoke and seldom drink, limit my artificial sweets, and appear healthy in that I'm not obese or noticeably overweight. They also know that I am jovial and not prone to long periods of depression and that I am a prolific writer and am seldom sick. Yet I suffered a stroke. It's one thing to watch a family member or close friend die or suffer from a disease, but it's a whole other thing when that same disease attacks your body. You don't know what it is to fight a disease until you do.

My trauma, the collective trauma of Black people, and the injustice of the health care system in America compels me to write my stroke memoir. In *The Source of Self-Regard*, Toni Morrison wrote, "Certain kinds of trauma visited on peoples are so deep, so cruel, that unlike money, unlike vengeance, even unlike justice, or rights, or the goodwill of others, only writers can translate such trauma and turn sorrow into meaning, sharpening the moral imagination."[1] Obviously, to tell one's trauma story, one must first survive. Tens of thousands of Black women suffer a stroke each year. Black women are 60 percent more likely to die of stroke than white women.

*Not Wanting* a *Thing to Be* the *Thing* is creative nonfiction, a stroke memoir written from my perspective as a Black woman, a biblical scholar, and a womanist writer. A womanist centers the experiences of Black women. Like Alice Walker's mother working in her flower garden, this book is the "work my soul must have."[2] I am a Black woman artist; I work with ideas and words, seldom with paint, but I'd like to paint more. Morrison wrote that the work of the Black artist is not a gift to the world; rather, it is a necessary endeavor. It is a necessary act. This memoir is my necessary act as a stroke survivor; it is my necessary story. I wrote this book because I am one of the tens of thousands of women and Black women who suffer stroke each year and survive. This is my fight story.

I write to provide an honest and vulnerable account of my stroke journey. While my recovery seems "amazing," as some have remarked, it has also been very difficult and is not over. When Dr. Renita Weems visited me in my home, she asked, "Is this the most difficult thing you've ever done?" I solemnly answered, "Yes, this is the most difficult thing I've ever done." Someone said to me in a Facebook post, "I'm thankful for your full recovery." While I truly appreciate the sentiment, it is not my story. I've never said or written that I've fully recovered. I'm not yet sure that "full recovery" is a thing. I live with invisible disabilities or body challenges. What people see is never all that a person is, particularly when it comes to physically

---

1. Morrison, *Source of Self-Regard*, ix.
2. Walker, *In Search of Our Mothers' Gardens*, 241.

challenged people. I write to put flesh on the bones of my stroke life and recovery journey.

Who am I enfleshed? First, I am Flora Ophelia Carson Smith's daughter. I am an educated African American cisgender woman. I am a biblical scholar trained at Howard University School of Divinity (master of divinity) and Harvard University (PhD, religion/New Testament). I am a progressive Christian, progressive in the sense that the religion I practice is not the same as the one into which I was indoctrinated. I no longer passively accept teachings, doctrines, and interpretations of biblical texts without critical reflection. I privilege the world in which we live as the more urgent context, as a sacred context, for engaging biblical texts. How we treat people and make them feel are more important than what we believe. I have published ten academic books. *Not Wanting a Thing to Be the Thing* is my first nonacademic book, and it's written for a much broader audience: for the Black community, women, poor people, and other communities disproportionately impacted by stroke and other preventable diseases.

I write because I am a walking miracle. I am an intergenerational miracle. Unless you know my family history, you don't know that I am also an intergenerational stroke survivor. I am an intergenerational miracle and survivor as a Black woman, going back as far as I know to my great-grandparents. My ancestresses survived enslavement; the era of lynching in America; Jim and Jane Crow; and anti-Black racial discrimination in housing, education, employment, and health care. Not all of my ancestors and ancestresses lived to see their late sixties, but they survived a lot of death-dealing situations and contexts, including those resulting from racism, sexism, and poverty perpetrated by America. Matthew Desmond writes the following in his book *Poverty By America*:

> Poverty is often material scarcity piled on chronic pain piled on incarceration piled on depression piled on addiction—on and on it goes. Poverty isn't a line. It's a tight knot of social maladies. It is connected to every social problem we care about—crime, health, education, housing—and its persistence in American life means that millions of families are denied safety and security and dignity in one of the richest nations in the history of the world.[3]

I write because I'm committed to social justice. I write to raise readers' consciousness about inequities in the US health care system and their impact on Black people who work within the system and Black bodies

---

3. Desmond, *Poverty by America*, 23.

that have no choice but to rely upon America's medical apartheid. African Americans have higher incidences and mortality rates of practically all major diseases, including cancer, heart disease, and stroke. We have a precarious relationship with America's health care system due to racism or racial bias, sexism, cost, and access. In *Just Medicine*, Dayna Bowen Matthew states that "the uncomfortable truth [is] that although overt racism, prejudice, and bigotry may have subsided in America, racial and ethnic injustice, unfairness, and even segregation in American health care have not. The most tragic proof that racial and ethnic injustice is alive and well is the phenomenon we politely call 'health care disparities,'" which are nothing more than toxic, preventable, and unjust implicit racial and ethnic biases.[4] It's still racism.

I write because too often our theologies of suffering and pain are problematic and harmful. They are easy and too-small Band-Aids applied to huge and complex wounds.

I write because I am an intergenerational creative. My ancestors and ancestresses created a life for themselves out of nothing or little of nothing. My great-grandparents George and Flora Jane Carson were born free and created a life together by often living apart so that each could go wherever they could find work, and they pooled their resources. They finally settled together in Cleveland, Tennessee, where they purchased a farm. Flora Jane became a nurse and helped found a hospital in Cleveland, Tennessee—a hospital that does not bear her name anywhere, as far as I know; that's what my mother told me. My mother's mother, Lillian Lay Carson of Cassville, Georgia, survived long enough to birth my mother and her three siblings, before dying of pneumonia when my mother was eight. My mother, Flora (February 4, 1929–2009), was born in Cassville, Georgia, grew up in Cleveland, Tennessee, and was raised by her grandparents. She became valedictorian of her high school graduating class and attended an HBCU (historically Black college or university) to become a nurse. My mother survived narcolepsy, polio, walking pneumonia, and two major strokes. The second stroke, nine years after the first, eventually took her life.

I am an intergenerational creative but not in the social media sense of the word. Mommy received an award as a first-class cook at the age of twenty-five, created or sketched a self-portrait with a pencil, planted an award-winning flower garden in front of our apartment in the projects, and resourcefully raised four children and a grandchild after being confined to

---

4. Matthew, *Just Medicine*, 2.

a wheelchair. My stroke story is necessarily connected with my mother's story. I write to tell the story of how my mother's story is interconnected with my own. Our stories overlap and diverge. My mother never wrote her story. I write to share pieces of her story through a daughter's womanist lens. Her story is and is not my story. Her story is a necessity too.

I recall a colleague, a Black woman, telling me when we were doctoral students at Harvard, "You are a fighter." Her comment gave me pause; I had never thought of myself in that way, had never used that word to describe myself. I reflected and realized that she was right. My mother—like most poor women, Black mothers, Black and Brown people, people generally living in poverty—was a fighter. I am also an intergenerational fighter, a warrior. This memoir is a creative act of necessity; it is also my fight story.

Every survivor's story is different *and* similar. But similarity is never sameness. And difference is contextual. Context is *the* difference. The human body, or embodiment, is context. The unique experiences of your body are context. Life experience is context. Your body is your body. Know your body. Family history is context. Theological formation is context. And so on. I write because my stroke story is unique and yet relatable, I hope.

I hope readers see *and do not* see themselves in my story. I hope readers think about their uniqueness and imagine themselves writing their own stories because somebody needs them. Writing one's story can be therapeutic for the writer and the communities for which they write. The wonderful prize-winning Nigerian poet Chimamanda Adichie states this about the danger of a single story: "Many stories matter; stories can be used to empower and humanize. They can be used to rob a people of their dignity, but they can also be used to repair. When we reject the single story, that there is never a single story about any place, [people, or experience], we regain a kind of paradise."[5] Diverse stories can expand our ability to empathize with different people and situations. Diverse stories expand our imagination and our arsenal for survival and thriving.

I hope this memoir will inspire other men and women, especially Black women, to write their stories. I hope it encourages readers to be resilient and to continue striving for wholeness. I hope this book is a poignant reminder that we are not alone; we stand on the shoulders of intergenerational survivors, creatives, and warriors. I hope you learn from my missteps and what I did right.

---

5. Adichie, "Danger of a Single Story."

# A Necessary Act

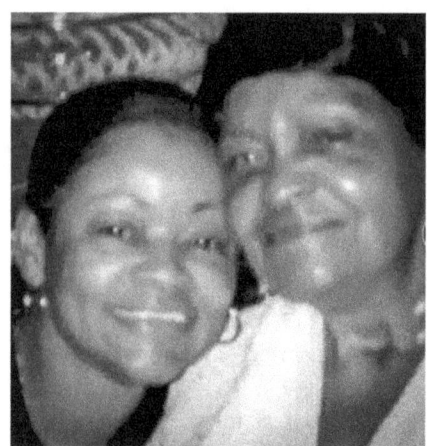
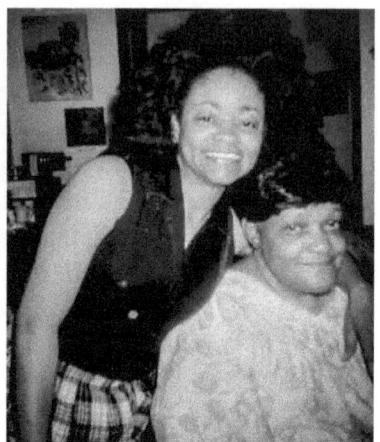
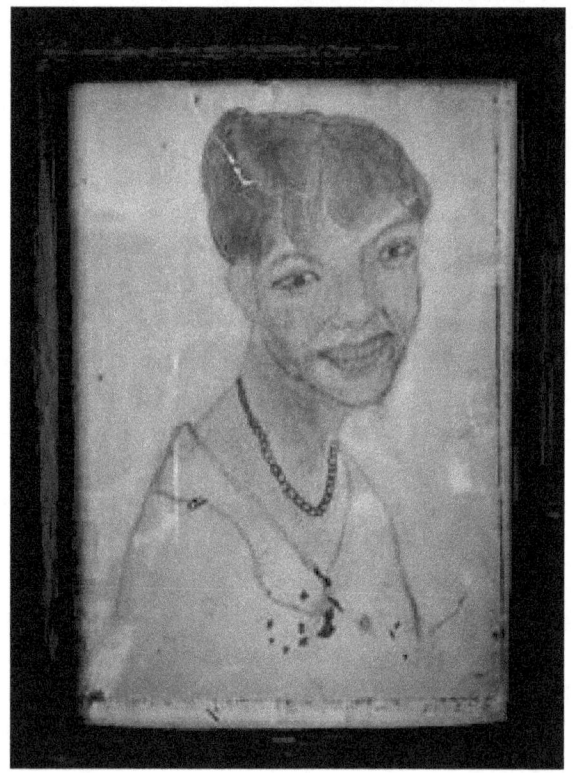

Part 1

# Not Wanting *a* Thing to Be *the* Thing Doesn't Make It Something Else

"Every criminal has a right to a lawyer, but we in America don't feel that every child has a right to a doctor." —Dr. Jocelyn Elders, Pediatrician, Professor of Pediatrics, and Former Surgeon General of the US from 1993–94

# 1

# I *Am* My Mother; I *Am Not* My Mother

HIDDEN UNDER THE SHORT black wig that framed her beautiful almost flawless ruddy brown-toned skin, except for a forgivable scar on her right cheek, was a rarely told story. The vertical mark tucked away in the fold of her skin when my mother, Flora, laughed was minimized by her perfectly set high cheek bones. It was the forgivable scar and proof that she had been in a car accident. It happened when she was a very young woman riding in the front passenger seat of a young man's car. The one scar that she concealed under her wigs was the first, initiating lifelong physical and emotional trauma—a rarely told story. Flora and her older sister Nellie wanted the same doll. Neither would let go, until Nellie did. Flora fell headfirst into the fireplace.

Flora had perfectly symmetrical, dark brown, almond-shaped eyes positioned about two inches below her brow line, straight white teeth (among the features I did not inherit), an inviting smile, and a heart-shaped face. My mother was beautiful and looked twenty years younger than her chronological age, but her body housed many scars. A scar is a story, often traumatic, needing to be heard. It's a story of struggle, not necessarily of defeat or victory but at least of survival. The older I become, the more I resemble my mother *and* Eartha Kitt, or so I've often been told. The Eartha comparisons started when I was eighteen years old. My mother looked nothing like Eartha Kitt. I am, and I am not, my mother. In health and in sickness, in youth and as I age, I *am* my mother. And I *am not* my mother.

Part 1: Not Wanting *a* Thing to Be *the* Thing Doesn't Make It Something Else

My mother's body bore scars, invisible to others, of struggle, survival, and resilience from the time she was a toddler through to her final years. Some scars last a lifetime.

After fifteen months, my body still bears postwar scars of my most life-changing struggle and trauma. Other than my medical records in the MyChart online portal, the marks on my body offer the only visible evidence of the struggle. The scars from three intravenous (IV) needles that nurses removed from my wrists and the inside folds of both my arms have mostly faded. A small, perfectly round brown scar raised in my flesh in the middle of my left wrist is proof that an IV needle once hung from my veins for weeks. Inaccessible to public view are the stubborn dark scars from the bruising to the left side of my lower stomach caused when the nurses plunged syringes into my belly to administer anticoagulants (blood thinners). Those dreaded shots tortured my body almost as much as the potassium drip that was once inserted in my right arm. On the lower right side of my stomach is a light, spotty scar from a blister that formed when a post-shot bandage was left on my stomach far too long. The only other noticeable (at least to me) scar mars my right baby finger, where I rested my eating utensils between that finger and the fold of my hand. My other fingers and thumb—swollen and creaseless from edema—were numb and less nimble. I couldn't balance a fork or spoon between my fingers to eat the way I had before war broke out in my body.

2

# Civil War

A COMPUTED AXIAL TOMOGRAPHY (CAT) scan and a magnetic resonance imaging (MRI) scan revealed that my body suffered three strokes (bleeding in or around the brain) or brain attacks in less than two months. According to the CAT scan, I suffered an "age-indeterminate left thalamic lacunar infarction, and an MRI of the brain showed an acute/subacute left infarct in the left side of the corpus callosum and a chronic lacunar infarct in the left thalamus." As I understand it, the lacunar infarct is a type of ischemic stroke (a life-threatening condition caused when blood clots or other blockages prevent blood flow to the brain) that affects deep brain structures. An ischemic stroke is often caused by high blood pressure or atherosclerosis (a disease of the arteries caused by deposits of plaques formed from fatty material on their inner walls). Blood vessels in my brain burst as blood coursed through them at too high a speed, causing the veins to narrow and blood to leak. The leaking blood vessels disrupted the flow of oxygen to my brain. Brain cells began dying immediately; consequently, parts of my body began malfunctioning. In addition to the hypertensive emergency, my sodium levels were too low; I had been washing and flushing the sodium from my body by drinking too much water.

The MRI cannot tell the doctors when I suffered the first two strokes; they are "age indeterminate" as previously noted. But reflecting back, I believe the first stroke occurred in early April 2023. I flew Delta from Atlanta to Washington, DC, on March 30 to attend the two-and-a-half-day annual meeting of the Society for the Study of Black Religion (SSBR). The next morning as I walk from my room in the conference hotel to the elevator, my muscles feel heavy and resistant.

Later that evening, as I sit for dinner at one of many round dining tables covered with bright white linen, a foreign, persistent pain pulsates in my upper left thigh. Under the tablecloth, I place my right hand on top of my left thigh and massage it in a downward motion, trying to soothe my body and relieve the throbbing. My body is temporarily consoled as I massage my left quadriceps femoris (the most voluminous muscle group in the human body). As soon as I stop, the throbbing resumes. For a split second, the idea of a stroke flashes into my mind. I dismiss it.

After finishing the tasty, tender roasted chicken breast and applauding the ending of the reenactment of a long phone dialogue between Martin Luther King Jr. and Robert F. Kennedy, I stand to leave the room. When I rise to my feet, the pain in my thigh abruptly stops. I lower the white flag of surrender to the idea that I'm having a stroke. Later, I feel as though the well-seasoned chicken breast has sunk like a rock to the bottom of my stomach where it lays all night, undigested. "I must be coming down with a virus," I soothe myself, settling for a less frightening self-diagnosis.

I do not yet know that a civil war has erupted in my body! Rebels attack loyalists; unionists fight against rogues! Through discomfort, abnormal sensations, and pain, my body tries warning me of the mutiny within.

# 3

# Terror

On April 2, 2023, the very morning that I return to Atlanta from DC, the warring members of my body agree upon a ceasefire and return to peaceful, normal operations. The truce allows me to maneuver the DC airport at my usual swift pace; sit and eat a healthy salad with Dr. Sheila Winborne, a sister-friend colleague from the Boston area, who had also attended the SSBR meeting; and board the plane to Atlanta. All of that normal activity confirms what I want to believe: *It's just a virus, and it's going away.*

However, once I'm home in Decatur, Georgia, my body rejects the once attractive salad; numbness and pain attack my feet and legs; fatigue and muscle weakness dog me. For almost a month, I continue to self-diagnose—*it must be a virus*! *It could not be a stroke. I don't want it to be a stroke! It is not a stroke. It's a virus.* So why don't I take a COVIDs test?

## The Thing Is

> Thing is
> not wanting a thing
> to be the thing
> doesn't make it
> something else.

The thing is, when you don't know what is wrong with you, that thing, whatever it is, terrorizes you. A guest on my *Beyond the Womanist Classroom* podcast, Dr. DeAnna Daniels, argues that when you cannot identify

Part 1: Not Wanting *a* Thing to Be *the* Thing Doesn't Make It Something Else

the thing that you fear, the thing that haunts you, that thing is a *terror*. Since you cannot identify it, you cannot do a thing about it. Once you can identify or name your terror, you can combat it. At that point it becomes *horror*. Horror is the thing you know, recognize, name, fight, and perhaps free yourself from.[1] Since you don't know what ails you, you are deceived when synchronization returns to your body, when your organisms and muscles agree on a temporary truce. *It's just a virus*, you convince yourself. Just a virus!? How soon you forget the many marked and unmarked graves COVID has dug—the disproportionate numbers of Black folk who have died unnecessarily.

*Just a virus?!* I console myself again. *This will pass!* I am relatively fit, especially for my age and considering my family history! I've geared up for this war most of my adult life. I live a better and healthier life than racism and sexism afforded my mother. I have better health insurance than I have ever had. So far I have avoided diabetes, the thing that plagued my mother and her sisters, ultimately killing them. Came close in 2020. Was on the cusp of a prediabetic diagnosis twice but pulled myself back from the brink. Panicked and frightened, I jumped into action. I began walking more often and tried to beat the Georgia heat by getting out to walk before 11:00 AM. My doctor at Morehouse Health said, "You need to walk every day." I reminded myself, as I have numerous times in my life, *You cannot bring ice cream and chocolate into the house! You will eat it!*

At home, I do the regular push-ups with my legs extended straight out behind me and arms straight and aligned with my shoulders. I've prided myself in being able to do twenty at a time and once worked my way to seventy-five in a day. I lift free weights. Once again, I join a fitness club and the YMCA. Jake and Abby Meyers recommend Black-owned Pinnacle Fitness, where they attend. Pinnacle focuses on weight or strength training. I even hire one of Pinnacle's personal trainers.

I live a more privileged and less stressful life than my mother did. She raised four children as a single-but-still-married parent, struggled with chronic and debilitating illnesses, never had adequate health care, and certainly didn't have the luxury of attending a fitness center. My mother, my two maternal aunts, and my brother died of strokes brought on by complications from diabetes. My maternal grandfather died from an aneurysm. As I've stated, my mother suffered two major strokes, nine years apart. I am determined not to be like my mother's father, my mother, or my aunts.

1. Smith, Beyond the Womanist Classroom podcast.

Neither Jamesina (Sina) nor Lenora, my sisters, have had a stroke. I am not having a stroke. Not in this regard. *I know it's just a virus.*

## Terror or Knowledge

The thing about terror
Is
Terror feeds on ignorance.
Terror thrives on not knowing.
Terror incapacitates.
Terror kills.
Willful or passive ignorance,
It doesn't matter.
The consequences, the damage
Are the same.
Don't be fooled into believing
That ignorance,
That not knowing,
Will permit you to avoid
To sidestep
The thing that terrorizes
And haunts you.
Avoidance is simply deferral
A deadly delay tactic,
Not a strategy.
You *cannot* avoid the thing that haunts you.
The thing that haunts you *is unavoidable*,
But you must know that unavoidable
Is not the same as unbeatable.
You need to know that unavoidable
Doesn't mean
You cannot survive the thing.
Knowing tells you what to fight.
Knowledge shows you how to fight.
Terror haunts us through ignorance
But knowing, knowledge
Deconstructs,
Incapacitates,
And perhaps, conquers
The thing that terrifies you.

# 4

# Stroke Symptoms in Women

A POST REPEATEDLY SHARED in the Facebook group Stroke Life Perspective lists three ways to recognize a brain attack with the acronym *FAST*: Face drooping, Arm weakness, Speech difficulty, which means Time to call an ambulance. Sometimes the acronym *BE* is added to the front of *FAST*: loss of Balance and Eye or vision changes. I experienced none of these symptoms.

Do you know that women can experience more subtle signs of stroke, as well as some symptoms in common with men? Common symptoms include weakness or numbness on one side of the face, weakness in the arms, trouble walking or sudden trouble with balance, slurred speech, and sudden vision loss. I had weakness in my arms and numbness in my hands and feet, but not in my face, and some trouble walking. Signs of stroke peculiar to women include dizziness; severe headache; significant fatigue; reduced swallowing reflex; loss of sensation in terms of smell, hearing, and taste; and shortness of breath or erratic heartbeat. I suffered significant fatigue, but not the other subtle symptoms. Women can experience general weakness, as I did. According to the American Heart Association's 2019 news report, women represent 60 percent of all stroke deaths because of subtle symptoms beginning with "fatigue, confusion, or general weakness as opposed to weakness on one side of the body."[1] I did not know that my fatigue and overall physical weakness constituted subtle signs of stroke in women. Researchers at the Ohio State University Wexner Center in Columbus,

---

1. American Heart Association News, "Is it Fatigue—or a Stroke?"

Ohio, surveyed a thousand women and found that only one in ten knew that hiccups together with unusual chest pain are an early warning sign of stroke in women. *Who imagined or knew? Certainly not I. I never imagined.* Some risk factors for stroke that are greater in women include lupus (which disproportionately impacts women, especially Black women), pregnancy, birth control pills, and hormone replacement therapy.

# 5

# It Might Be a Stroke

I CANNOT SECURE AN emergency appointment with my primary care doctor for a couple of weeks. Evidently, many doctors no longer offer their patients emergency appointments. So, in choosing to wait for an appointment with my primary care doctor, I miss another opportunity to visit the hospital emergency room (ER). I will not see my primary care doctor until 3:00 PM on Monday, May 1, 2023. Dr. Moss (not her actual name) is a Black middle-aged woman of African descent. A colleague recommended her. When I first met Dr. Moss, she was excited to learn that I teach at a seminary. She confided that she dreams of attending seminary when she retires.

At Dr. Moss's office, my blood pressure reads 220/110. In a calm, slow, low voice and with a deeply concerned facial expression, Dr. Moss asks, "How did you get here?"

"I drove."

"You don't feel dizzy? Are you having headaches?"

"No, I only feel pain in my left arm."

I experience no noticeable change in my facial expression; it doesn't droop on one side. I can see that Dr. Moss feels badly for me. She orders an electrocardiogram (EKG), which shows that my heart is fine; it is beating normally. I haven't suffered a heart attack. I am relieved, but only for a few brief seconds. Dr. Moss raises the possibility that I have suffered a stroke. I weep uncontrollably. When she places her arm around my shoulders, I weep even more. I think when people show compassion, we feel it is safe to be fully vulnerable. Dr. Moss shares that her husband suffered a stroke as the result of COVID. "But he's alright now. He recovered fully," she says. I take some comfort in knowing her husband recovered. I am prescribed 10 mgs of carvedilol phosphate once a day. "A higher dosage could lower your blood pressure more rapidly but might cause you to feel worse," she explains. Dr. Moss thinks she has some carvedilol samples on hand that she could give me but discovers that she no longer has them. A prescription for the carvedilol is sent to my pharmacy, which I pick up on my way home. "If your condition worsens, you should go to the ER." It gets worse, but I avoid the ER.

# 6

# Urgent Care

Exhausted and terrified, on May 12, 2023, I Google the urgent care nearest to me. The Piedmont Urgent Care on Ponce de Leon Avenue in Atlanta is only a few miles away. After a relatively short wait (when you are in enough pain, no wait is brief), an African American nurse greets me and escorts me to an exam room where she weighs me and takes my blood pressure. Shockingly, my blood pressure reads 176/99! I tear up from the inside out. The carvedilol my primary care doctor prescribed has helped, but it's not enough.

Some minutes after the nurse leaves me alone in the exam room, a relatively young male doctor, who looks like he is of South Asian, perhaps Indian origins, enters the room. Frightened and eager for answers and a solution that might put me on the path back to wellness, I tell him about the lack of energy, fatigue, and numbness and pain in my feet, and I also relate that I vomited, but only once, the day I returned from DC. The doctor demonstrates no real concern or empathy for my deteriorating condition. He taps my knees with a little rubber hammer and announces that my reflexes are fine. *But my feet and toes are numb! And I feel awful! Something is terribly wrong!*

The urgent care doctor exits the room so that he might "think about" my symptoms, he says. When he returns after about five minutes, he informs me that he has no idea what is wrong with me. Evidently, he too is unaware of the presenting symptoms of stroke in women. He dismisses me, rather quickly, despite a blood pressure reading of 176/99. He prescribes medication for nausea and a recommendation to see a neurologist; the latter he writes on the visit summary but doesn't bother to verbalize to me during the actual visit. I feel unseen and unheard. I am in and out of urgent care very quickly. Ironically, I am avoiding the ER partly out of fear of a too-long waiting period during which time my condition would worsen and I could die. But quick access does not amount to excellent or compassionate care.

As I leave the urgent care exam room, my tired, glassy, and disappointed eyes meet and momentarily lock with the sympathetic stare of the young African American nurse who is sitting at the desk adjacent to the exam room. She is the nurse who took my blood pressure and knows it is dangerously elevated. Perhaps she is warning me, without words, with her dark brown compassionate eyes: "Ma'am, you are in real bad shape; you need an immediate intervention. Unfortunately, these folks are not helping you." I am released to unresolved suffering.

Later that day or the next, I search the internet for the urgent care doctor, and I discover Yelp reviewers had similar experiences with him. They feel he did not seem to care. I do not know the race or ethnicity of those reviewers, so I don't know for certain that his lack of compassion was the result of anti-Black racism. But I do know from experience and statistics that Black patients are treated less compassionately by the health care system and by white doctors.[1]

A few days later, I miss a call from Piedmont Urgent Care. An African American woman leaves a phone message: "Ms. Smith, we are just checking to see if you are okay." I guess that is something. I don't return the call. What else can I tell them? What else do they need to know? They know that I am not okay! The urgent care doctor confirmed my worst fears about the health care system's callous, careless doctors. In retrospect, the urgent care doctor should have sent me to the ER. I should have known and done better. Would I live to know better? If I live, in what physical conditional will I survive?

If I didn't know other South Asian or Indian people, I might be tempted to think that they are all anti-Black racists who lack compassion for Black people. Intellectually, I know that no one person (or a few) ever represents a whole people. I know plenty of non-Black people hold negative stereotypes about Black people and are curious about Black people, about

---

1. Alcindor et al., "History of Abuse in American Medicine"; Bridges, "Implicit Bias and Racial Disparities in Health Care."

their hair among other stuff. I once traveled to Bangalore, India, to dialogue with colleagues about the Dalit struggle and the civil rights struggle among African Americans. I remember standing in a crowded alley listening to a poor Dalit woman tell her story of struggle under the caste system in India, when I felt something in my natural hair. I turned to find that it was not *something* but some*one*'s fingers in my hair. One of my Indian colleagues, who was more intrigued by my hair than by the woman's story, took it upon herself to grope my natural hair. I felt violated and indignant but didn't permit myself to show it. I did not want to disrupt the Dalit woman's story, to disrespect her; she and her neighbors had experienced enough of that.

Later that day, a different Indian colleague asked me if she could touch my hair. At least she didn't take the liberty of touching my body without my permission. I was in Bangalore with some Black scholars to dialogue about what Dalits might learn from the African American struggle in the US. I learned that some of my Indian colleagues felt that we have nothing to teach them.

The urgent care doctor is similar and different from my New Testament (NT) colleague at the seminary where I teach, Dr. Raj Nadella. Raj is a caring human being. His father died in India; his mother still lives there. Raj often checks on me during my illness. I will say more about Raj and his wife, Amy, later.

# 7

# Showing Up

Neither my symptoms nor my attendance in class changes in April and May of 2023. I don't miss a single day of my New Testament Interpretation (NTI) class that meets at 8:30 on Tuesday and Friday mornings for an hour and a half. I do cancel one session of my Dissent course, which also convenes Tuesdays but from 6:30 to 8:30 in the evening. It is a long teaching day. I try to prepare for both classes on Mondays so that I can nap or rest between the two classes the following day. Nevertheless, because of fatigue, I *sit* through each class session with reduced strength and vitality. Before I became sick, I would stand, pace in the space in front of the room, share a PowerPoint presentation, and lecture for roughly an hour. I usually talk with my arms and hands as well as my voice. Regardless of how I'm feeling, though, I never lecture for long stretches of time; I prefer informed dialogue with students. According to Paulo Freire, liberative education is dialogical, and teachers are teacher-students while students are student-teachers. We learn from one another; we bring our pre-knowledges and experiences into the classroom.

The Dissent class is small; each student is required to lead discussion of assigned readings twice during the semester. For the first time in my teaching career, an assignment in both courses requires students to respond creatively to one of the assigned readings for each week. For example, students can write poetry or draw pictures. The few students in the Dissent course don't get it at first; they think "creative response" means the response of a creative (such as Maya Angelou) rather than a response they create themselves. A sick teacher is an impatient teacher, but not necessarily an unreasonable one. I bear responsibility for this misunderstanding.

On the other hand, the NTI students flourish with the creative assignment. They respond to readings with original drawings and inventions, poetry, short essays, and collages. For example, an African American woman student, Dr. Montisa, collects diverse pairs of eyeglasses, ties a string to each, and attaches them to a wooden stick like a wind chime to demonstrate how readers bring various contextual lenses to the task of biblical interpretation. Moved by a course reading about social justice, an African American woman student, Jonique, writes a poem entitled "My Brothers' and Sisters' Keeper." The first line reads, "When did we forget to treat our neighbor as ourselves?" and the poem culminates with "Inaction is compliance by another name that lends a foul stench to the nostrils and proclaims, 'better them than me.'" Jordan, a white male student in his late twenties to early thirties with a teddy-bear-like frame, creates a reflection entitled "Sassy" in response to my essay about Black women's sass and talk-back and the Syrophoenician woman's encounter with Jesus in Mark's Gospel. Jordan writes,

> I find myself wondering what sassy behavior looks like for a cisgendered man . . . I am taking time, even if it is for an assignment, to simply let my thoughts flow . . . which I find difficult to do. Sometimes I allow my own perceptions to gaslight me into doing things I do not want to do . . . I feel the truly sassy thing to do is to find a humble way of expressing sassiness. A way of occupying space in which I never deny who I am, and yet am conscious of the needs and desires of others. Even thinking about this makes me feel at peace.

The students bring to the classroom an energy that I lack; they encourage my spirit. Part of me shows up for them and vice versa. I approach Dr. Spurrier, the associate dean of worship life, about allowing space for the NTI students to share their creative responses in chapel. She welcomes the idea and suggests they do this during a Wednesday noon prayer hour. Enthusiastically, the students create a visual display using a metal coat rack about six feet long and three feet wide on which they hang, with clothes pins, their select creations. Despite how badly I've been feeling those last two months, the students thrive. It says a lot for a good syllabus and student enthusiasm.

## Showing Up

On Friday morning, May 5, 2023, in the last session of the NTI course and in the final few minutes of the course, I sob uncontrollably. I am relieved that we made it to the end of the semester. I am also afraid because my condition is not improving. But now I can stop showing up and performing. I can rest and focus on the upheaval in my body. Much later, I would have a phone conversation with Dr. Lynne Westfield, the director of the Wabash Center for Teaching and Learning, about the creative writing workshop I was selected to attend in July 2023. At some point in our conversation, Lynne says "Women, and particularly Black women, just keep showing up. We don't stop and take care of ourselves." Sadly, it is true.

In those final minutes, my wonderful, compassionate, and creative NTI students pray for and cry with me. Jordan approaches. "Dr. Smith, can I hug you?" Through my tears, I say "Yes." And he does. That is the first but not the last hug I receive from Jordan.

Hugs are therapeutic. Experts say humans need hugs daily. According to Christine Comaford, hugs strengthen our immune system and balance our bodies. They "increase circulation and help balance our sympathetic (fight/flight/freeze) and parasympathetic (regulates rest and digest activities) nervous systems."[1] Hugs also remind us that we are not alone, that we belong, and that we are being seen and matter to someone, all of which can increase self-esteem. Comaford suggests that, if we need more hugs, we should ask for hugs and hug ourselves.[2] Unfortunately, we often find it easier to tear ourselves down rather than embrace and speak kindly to ourselves. When we know better, we must do better.

I am thankful for the physical and verbal hugs that my students gift me. Students in my Dissent course suggest—alright, practically insist—on two occasions that I visit the ER. I dismiss their caring and wise advice. Unfortunately, the idea of visiting the ER scares me more than not knowing for certain what is happening in my body. *Why am I not listening to my students?* I wish I had listened on the very day they insisted that I go to the ER. But I can't bring myself to accept that I am seriously ER-level ill. I can't yet face the terror of the war within.

As I look back at the calendar I keep in my iPhone, I'm amazed at the meetings—admissions, faculty development, executive committee of the faculty, faculty business, faculty teaching, Bible Area—that I was expected to and pushed myself to attend, despite being unwell. We cannot always

---

1. Comaford, "Are You Getting Enough Hugs?"
2. Comaford, "Are You Getting Enough Hugs?"

perform as expected; institutions will carry on without us. To a small degree, I dissent, refusing to attend what I feel are overbearing admissions committee meetings, and I miss a faculty meeting (we have two a month) for the first time since my hire in July 2019. To be fair, I told the academic dean, Christine Yoder, on several occasions, "I'm getting better." Part of me believes or wants to believe that my health is improving as the symptoms shift from the right to the left side of my body and back again. I don't know I am experiencing strokes on both sides of my brain as a result of "grossly high blood pressure," which proves too much for parts of my body to bear without erupting into a full-blown civil war.

## 8

# The ER
## I Can't Write My Name

THE WORST AND LAST stroke strikes around two o'clock in the morning on May 24, 2023. I am home alone, but not solitary in my body. Pain envelops me. I awaken to unbearable agony in my right leg.

I remember when my mother, Flora, declined her doctor's suggestion that she consider knee replacement surgery—it was highly experimental in the late 1960s and early 1970s. She refused to be "anybody's guinea pig." My mother told my siblings and me that she preferred the pain of a living joint to a dead one. Her fears were not unfounded or unreasonable. In her book *Medical Apartheid*, Harriet Washington recounts the painful, dehumanizing history of gynecological experimentation that J. Marion Sims, the father of modern gynecology, performed on enslaved Black girls' bodies for the benefit of white women's survival and health.[1] Some things do not change. Racism, sexism, classism, queerphobia, and transphobia are forms of violence that impact Black well-being and health. Donna Christian-Christensen, MD, former chair of the Congressional Black Caucus Health Braintrust, asserts that "health disparities are the civil rights issue of the 21st century."[2]

Pain is our friend; it is one of the body's warning signals. Ignoring the body's pain is like siding with the enemy. My body is screaming so intensely,

---

1. Washington, *Medical Apartheid*.
2. Washington, *Medical Apartheid*, 3.

## Part 1: Not Wanting *a* Thing to Be *the* Thing Doesn't Make It Something Else

like a wounded soldier alone in the dead of night in a shadowy forest in enemy territory. I can no longer ignore her high-pitched unrelenting cries as they echo through my body and disrupt the silence of my bedroom and the moonlit darkness that crept into the house.

Extra-strength Tylenol PM does not console or anesthetize my pain. That third stroke and the suffering it ignites forces me into the ER and the Intensive Care Unit (ICU). Neither the ER nor the ICU can halt the damage that the strokes have put in motion.

The two emergency medical technicians (EMTs) or paramedics in the ambulance who respond to my 911 call ask what hospital I would like them to deliver me to. I respond, "The closest one." Emory Hospital (EH) in Decatur is about two to three miles away from my home. But it has no empty beds that night. The ride to EH in Atlanta took a bit longer. When you are in crisis and experiencing pain like the pain my mother once described as "I didn't know it was humanly possible," a bit longer feels much too long.

When I think of the ER, I envision extremely long waiting periods; silent suffering; insensitive, overworked health care professionals; and certain death. I wish someone had told me that the ER can be the lesser of two evils, the greater evil being an assemblage of not knowing, denial, assuming you know what you really don't know, and the fear of confronting the terror of one's family medical history. In fact, I wish I had known that the ER is not an evil at all. The evil is the illness (not the sick person). The evil is racism and other isms. The evil is underfunded health care systems. The evil is the refusal to acknowledge the implicit biases of health workers so as to exorcise these biases and their harmful and fatal impact on patients.

I learned to hate and fear ERs because of the many times that I accompanied my mother to an ER where she suffered while waiting to be seen and where, too often, she wasn't treated very well. I knew it as a frigid space where people deteriorated and could be discharged without proper treatment and sent home to die.

In that frigid ER space, I begin my journey to better health. It begins with knowing the terror within that haunts through the bloodline. In that space I most wanted to avoid, the EMTs, two late twenties to early thirtyish men, one Black (the EMT who treated me in the ambulance) and the other Caucasian (the ambulance driver), guide me on a gurney into a space both familiar and unfamiliar to me. They are my angels.

I have been here in this space before but not in this ailing body and not in this hospital in this state and city. I had accompanied my mother too many times. Now, strangers accompany me. If I remember correctly—pain can dull the memory—the two men wear dark blue short-sleeve cotton shirts with matching trousers. They work in tandem and both treat me with compassion and care.

EH in Atlanta on Clifton Road doesn't have space in the ICU or the hospital either. But perhaps it is the one most likely to have a bed sooner rather than later. That's where my two EMT friends park me on the gurney. And I am glad I landed there, for the most part.

Vacant desks are spaced around a wide tile path. One, two, or at most three women and men dressed in white or light blue uniforms stand, convene, or scamper through the relatively empty, dull white area of the ER. It would be another hour before I see another nurse and before an empty bed becomes available in the ICU. Hospitals everywhere are experiencing personnel shortages, particularly of nurses. Do you know that the nursing shortage has hit Georgia especially hard? The state is anticipated to experience the second-worst shortage nationwide over the next ten years. Because of low wages and high stress, nurses are exiting Georgia or forsaking the vocation entirely. If the environment is not safe for nurses, what about the patients? Angelic and perhaps not so angelic health care workers are charged with my care. I will introduce you to them, one by one.

Behind me sit and stand my two alert and friendly EMT angels, patiently waiting for me to be treated. Are they also concerned that this is taking so long? Are they wondering if I will survive? In what condition will I survive? Above me hovers a lighted flat ceiling. I'm surrounded by walls with sad and miraculous stories to tell, if they could speak.

I expected the ER to be bustling. Instead, as far as I can see and imagine, it is like the aftermath of a war zone: sparse and silent. The opening scene from the postapocalyptic film *The Book of Eli* comes to mind. It's around three in the morning in the ER; it's the NOC shift (from the Latin word *noctis* meaning night; 11:00 PM to 7:00 AM). The night isn't sequestered outside; it seeps into all human-made structures, into hospitals and homes. After all, the night is the original primordial thing or element. The artificial light in the ER mitigates the night. Still, the ER is morbidly silent, not because of the night; it's the threat and nearness of death. The ER is practically empty, with side pockets of offices and rooms where I imagine a scant number of night-shift technicians, phlebotomists, interns, doctors, and nurses perform their necessary duties of patient care and mutual support. They do their work within a counterintuitive timeframe—when the human body demands sleep or rest to maintain health—and they do it for the sake of other people's health. I envision patients with tubes plugged into their veins, struggling to sleep. But they suffer from insomnia, more obviously, due to excruciating pain, anxiety, or both, unless a nurse has administered a doctor-approved painkiller as potent as oxycodone. From my experience, Tylenol PM is as impotent as an 81 mg baby aspirin when the body or mind is fighting or overcome with anxiety—or a stroke.

My two EMT friends and I are the sole audience at this drive-in movie theater. I'd rather be watching Denzel Washington on the big screen than being the star of my own internecine war story or postapocalyptic film. I'm not having an out-of-body experience; my body knows, intimately feels, the trauma of the civil war within.

When two hospital workers enter the stage at once and engage one another, they speak in whispers. Or maybe they are standing so far from me I cannot hear them well? Or does my pain interfere with my hearing? I am the only one of three audience members who is stretched out on a reclined seat. I'm losing the battle to stifle my pain. My body intermittently releases minor and major groans. The other actors in this space are accustomed to such audience participation. God knows, Black people in a movie theater cannot resist talking back to the characters in a film, as if the actors can hear us. I hate how women are portrayed as stupid in movies, especially when being chased by a murderer or rapist. So we shout at the screen, "Why did you just run into the woods where there's nobody to help you?" "Why did she run onto the darkest, emptiest street she could find?" "Are you crazy?" "What the heck!" The actors, the ones in the ER, ignore me, until the script demands that they interact with me.

## I Can't Sign My Name

After what feels like an eternity, an ER nurse approaches me and puts a pen in my right hand. All my life I have been right-handed. The nurse holds the hospital admittance form attached to a clip board in front of me to sign. But my right hand does not understand what my brain is asking it to do. My cerebrum resorts to treating my right hand like a young soldier in training, teaching her to decipher and respond to the instructions that her commanding officer is belting out. My brain tries communicating with my hand but in language that has become foreign to it: *Touch the paper. Touch the paper. Touch the paper with the pen. Touch the paper with the pen.*

Repetition is sometimes ineffective nagging, but not in this moment. After the longest couple of minutes, my hand understands what my brain is saying. My hand touches pen to paper. But then the connection fails at the point of contact, the way a cell phone connection drops when you drive under a bridge or upon entering remote rural and poorer areas of the world without access to broadband due to cost, availability, or both. My right hand does not remember how to behave in this moment; it doesn't know how to sign my name. The connection is damaged. Part of me wants to sign my name, but the connection is lost. I–cannot–write–my–name! I–cannot–write–my–name! I'm shocked. I watch in slow-motion terror the struggle within my body play out in front of me. Fear and hopelessness threaten to consume me. The nurse prompts me to make a mark. I can hear and understand her. That's a good sign. I eventually manage to scribble something, to make a mark, but nothing that comes close to resembling the letters *M*, *S*, or my name.

## No Too Sick to Be Gracious

After "signing" the admittance papers, the waiting resumes. I can't see them—the other three to four people waiting in agony for beds in the ICU. They are further along in the admissions process. I do not encounter any other ER patients until they roll me to the interior space of the ER to have blood drawn. Two people precede me in that space, waiting for their blood to be drawn. When my time arrives, a young, attractive African American woman draws my blood but not before she gleefully compliments me, almost like a fan to a celebrity. "You look much younger than your age," she says. "I hope to look as good as you when I am your age." I reply, "Thank you!" I'm not too sick to be gracious. Sickness can make you feel older than you are. My body gracefully and gratefully digests her generous words; they momentarily rally my cells and warm my body in that frigid space. She gifted me a very brief reprieve from the effects of the long wait, which has dragged on unbearably and unnecessarily in my view, between our arrival in the ER and my finally reaching her dedicated space. Chronic pain and sickness can also mature you, physically, emotionally, and spiritually. And it can have the opposite effect.

# 9

# Quadruple Risk

IF YOU HAVE A family history of stroke and are Black, it is unlikely you can avoid a stroke. The question is how debilitating it will be. A family history of stroke, as well as race, gender, and age—all considered "uncontrollable" risk factors of stroke—together with the development of extremely high blood pressure (a controllable risk factor), made me an excellent candidate for a stroke.[1] It is a wonder that I hadn't suffered a stroke sooner. I like to think I had been doing some things right, but I could have done better. People of all ages suffer strokes, but the older we are, the greater the risk. Women over their lifetimes suffer more strokes than men. And Black and Hispanic people have a higher risk because they have high blood pressure at greater rates than other races. Sexism is stressful. Racism is a stressor.

Of course, a family history of stroke increases your risk. As I said, my maternal grandfather died of an aneurysm. My mother suffered two major strokes nine years apart; the last one eventually resulted in her death in 2009. My brother developed adult-onset diabetes in his late fifties. In 2022, he died after suffering a stroke during the COVID crisis. A few weeks before I ended up in the ER, I remember calling my sister, Sina—who's older by a year and some months—and telling her how bad I felt. She quickly said, "You know it could be a stroke. Papa died of an aneurysm and Mom of a major stroke." I dismissed her opinion as pessimistic. *Sina is always wallowing in negativity*, I told myself. Which context—family history or Sina's perceived negativity—would I allow to inform my behavior? I am

---

1. American Stroke Association, "Let's Talk About Risk Factors of Stroke."

always telling my biblical studies students that *context is everything* when interpreting texts. We choose what contexts to privilege and which ones to ignore. You might choose to ignore what you already know. You might elect to prioritize the more agreeable context and render invisible the less pleasant context, the one that doesn't fit your doctrinal commitments or ideological biases. The unpleasant fact that you don't know or choose not to recognize when it confronts you can injure or kill you. As a sixty-five-year-old Black woman whose mother and maternal grandfather suffered debilitating and fatal strokes, I had four strikes against me—age, race, gender, and family history. Stroke was a quadruple threat.

Yet, a person can suffer a stroke at any age in an otherwise healthy body with good blood sugar and cholesterol levels. A seventeen-year-old healthy African American girl suffered seven strokes after a fall, her mother would tell me as I sat in the waiting room of the outpatient therapy clinic, months after my initial ER visit. You could be that person who exercises routinely, drinks plenty of water, eats healthily 80 to 90 percent of the time, meditates, maintains a positive view of life, laughs a lot, devotes time to spiritual practices, and so on, and you could still have a stroke.

# 10

# They Don't Serve Food in the ICU

THE NIGHT I CALLED 911, the two Black EMTs who arrived first (before the ambulance) asked, "Can you walk to the ambulance?" I replied, "Yes, I think I can walk." Despite my pain, I remained independent. I was still mobile. It meant things weren't as bad as I felt. I walked slowly from my home and stepped into the ambulance parked at the curb in front of my house.

On my first day in the ICU, I remember laying in the bed for a long time before seeing a nurse or doctor again. I do not yet have a hospital gown. Despite being fully clothed in my street clothes, my body shivers from the icy-cold air conditioning, and I badly need to use the bathroom. I call out for assistance as loudly as I can, several times. Nobody responds or hears me. The few people on duty are assigned more than a normal quota of patients. When I feel that my bladder is about to burst if I wait any longer, I slowly roll myself off the bed and stumble into the hallway where I ask a random man, "Can you tell me where the bathroom is?" He points the direction. I stay close to the wall, sometimes hugging it with one hand and balancing my body with the other hand. I arrive at the bathroom without falling down. After I empty my bladder, I return to the bed on the same path and in the same manner. Clearly, my body has weakened, but I can still walk.

Back in the bed, I'm freezing. The ICU rooms are cubicles with curtains serving as the door between me and the hallway traffic. But all is quiet. Traffic is slow and sometimes nonexistent. When a nurse finally enters my room, I tell her that I am freezing and ask for extra blankets. She asks if I would like a "warming blanket." "Yes, please," I say, having no idea what a warming blanket is, but it sounds good. The nurse returns with a very toasty blanket, as though it had come fresh out of a hot dryer. After a while, I also realize that I have not eaten in a long time.

Laying in my ICU bed, starving, I confide to God, *If this is it, I'm ready to die.* Eventually a nurse appears to help me change from my street clothes into a hospital gown. She wipes my body down and places two IVs (intravenous lines) into the veins of my left arm, one at my wrist and one inside the fold of my elbow.

"I am really hungry. I haven't eaten since yesterday morning," I tell the nurse.

"We don't have food in the ICU."

*You must be kidding!* I think to myself.

"I will see if I can find something for you to eat," she says.

But first they must make sure that I can swallow solid foods without choking. Who knew that hospitals don't serve food in the ICU?! Not me! The boundary line between the ER and ICU is blurry to me.

Before arriving in the ER and ICU, I have already lost a fifth of my body weight. I've been suffering at home, not able to stand on my feet long enough to prepare home-cooked meals. I resort to Instacarting items like canned soup, cottage cheese, yogurt, fruit, and Amy's Kitchen frozen meals. Sometimes I order meals through DoorDash but prefer not too; they're so salty.

After some hours, the ICU nurse scrounges up some soft food, a sort of tasteless applesauce; it's certainly not Mott's. The food they serve me encourages fasting and not feasting. I eat what I can stomach. Eventually, the amount of liquids I am allowed to drink is limited because my sodium levels are low. I don't recall but think at some point they start feeding me some nutrients intravenously.

## 11

# Fight

SOME PEOPLE BELIEVE THAT our bodies betray us when we fall prey to diseases and illnesses. But I have allies within and outside my body, fighting with me. During my short stay in the ICU, a kind nurse, an angel, sympathetically and compassionately encourages me to fight for my survival. She gently advises, "Your recovery will depend on your attitude." Her words light a tiny spark in me. As the song goes, *It only takes a spark to get a fire going*. I am still here; this must not be the end. It is not the end, until it is. I must join the fight for my survival. Parts of my body are fighting to survive because I am still here. While cells in my brain are dying as it hemorrhages, other cells remain alive and are fighting for me. Step one toward survival and recovery: Pick a side in this war. Today, I choose to fight *with* my body and not against it.

### Fight

On this day,
At this hour,
In this moment,
I choose to fight
With my body.
My body and I
We choose life.
Parts of me are dying.
And parts of me live.

Fight

Life and death co-exist
In this body.

12

# My Mother Was a Nurse; I Wanted to Be Like Her

IN 1948, MY MOTHER earned her home nursing certificate from Morristown Normal Industrial College, a historically Black school supported by the Episcopal Methodist Church. My mother was the first and most compassionate nurse I have known. The Trent sisters, two elderly white women, lived in the same projects as us in Columbus, Ohio; they could call my mother when they needed assistance, and she'd go see about them. Before she lived in Columbus, Mommy resided in Cleveland, Ohio where she worked at St. Luke's Hospital. She often told the story of how she held an elderly patient's hand as death rattled in his throat and he took his last breath, which "sliced through my body like an ice-cold knife." Mom believed in "treating patients like they are my own parents." Her mother died when she was about eight years old; her grandparents raised her and her sister Nellie in Cleveland, Tennessee. When (great-) Grandma Flora died, Mom traveled to Cleveland and brought great-grandfather Daddy George to live with us in our two-bedroom apartment in the housing projects in Columbus. Mom gave her bed to Daddy George until he died. I, Sina, and Fred shared the other bedroom. When I was a teenager, my mother, who had been in a wheelchair since I was ten years old, would make and serve me hot tea with a dose of Midol whenever excruciating menstrual pains forced me to curl up in a fetal position in bed for at least a day.

In my twenties, when I lived in Takoma Park, Maryland, I signed up to be a "candy striper"; I wanted to be like my mother. Women who were trained to be hospital volunteers back then wore pink-and-white–striped uniforms. While serving as a candy striper at Washington Adventist Hospital, I was asked to assist a nurse in administering an enema, but this nauseated novice fled the hospital room. I can change hospital bedding, clothe a patient, and shave a patient, but I draw the line at enemas. However, when your mother becomes the patient, you will do the thing that, as a candy striper, you could not do for a stranger.

As noted, I was about ten years old when my mother lost the ability to walk and had to use a wheelchair. I deeply loved and greatly admired my mother. My older sister teased that, when Mommy died, they'd have to put me in the coffin too. But twice in my life—when I developed sciatica and after my stroke—I feared being in the same debilitating physical condition as my mother. Both times, I feared losing my ability to walk. Would I become the thing I feared? Or would hope, self-determination, personal effort, health care workers, prayers, and God intervene to overcome the horror?

Part 1: Not Wanting *a* Thing to Be *the* Thing Doesn't Make It Something Else

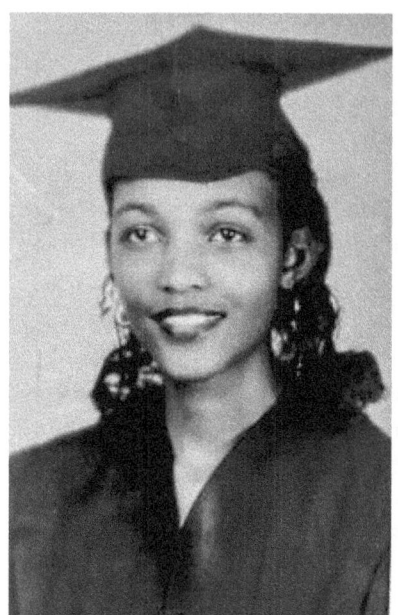
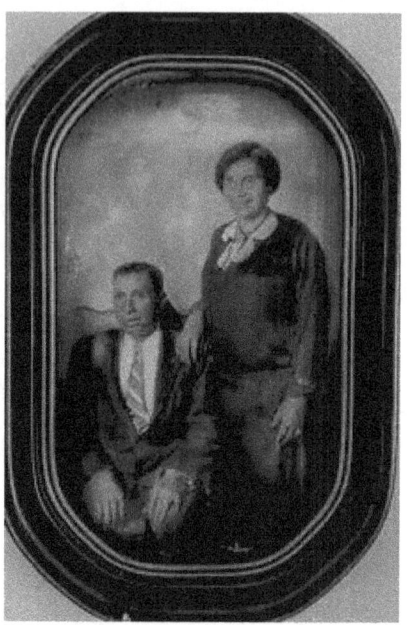
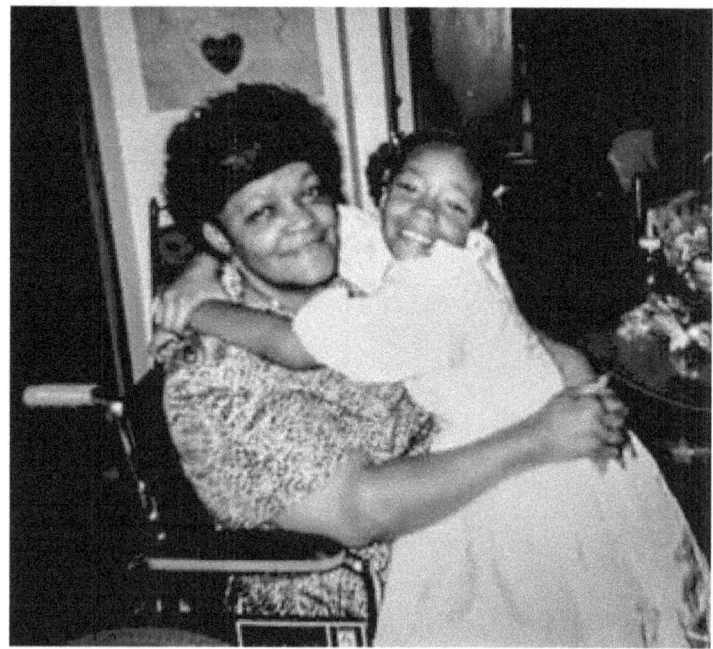

## 13

# Not On My Watch

IN THE ICU, I lack the bandwidth to respond to text messages or phone calls from people, including some family members, about my condition. Heck, I'm still learning about the status of my health and coming to terms with the information that the doctors and nurses share with me. Relatives and friends who have my cell phone number text, "How are you?" I know they all mean well and are concerned, but it annoys me that they should expect me to respond from the ICU and after suffering a stroke! I *feel* like responding, "How do you think I am after suffering a stroke?!" but I refrain. I'm overwhelmed. I cannot respond, but not because I cannot speak or think. My brain is traumatized, and my entire body has been impacted. The damage has yet to be assessed; deterioration has not ceased.

I have no close family members nearby. Dr. Lisa Weaver, a sister-friend, Black woman, neighbor, and colleague decisively vows, "I will not let a Black woman suffer alone. Not on my watch." At the time, Lisa, Dr. Marcia Riggs, and I are the three Black women faculty members at Columbia Theological Seminary (CTS), which is a predominantly white and Presbyterian institution of higher education. We check on each other, share meals together, commiserate, and support each other as necessary. Lisa asks, "Who do you want me to contact for you? What do you want me to tell them? If you can give me names and numbers, I'll let them know how you are doing from day to day." Lisa calls the ICU and visits Emory regularly to check on my progress; she brings me clothes and other personal items and is kind enough to inform Christine Yoder and other colleagues and friends, as well as some of my relatives, of my condition and progress. My two sisters, Sina and Lenora, and my oldest niece Misty call Emory from Columbus, Ohio, and ask about my condition, but most of the time Lisa updates them so that I'm not more overwhelmed than I already am. I'm grateful.

# 14

# From ICU to a Bed in EH

I'M UNCERTAIN IF EMORY ICU and Emory Hospital (EH) are two separate institutions, but my hospital notes in MyChart conflate the two. When I entered Emory's ICU on May 24, MyChart states that I actually entered EH. But I am not given a bed at EH for a few days. It's strange that, before writing this memoir, I would tell people that I was in Emory's ICU for two or three days, and maybe I was. But MyChart doesn't make the same distinction between Emory ICU and EH. My admission date to Emory ICU is therefore recorded as being the same as my admittance to EH; there is no boundary line in the records. Only in my mind.

Nevertheless, eventually, with the right cocktail of drugs, the Emory ICU doctors and nurses successfully lower my blood pressure so that it is no longer *grossly* high, though it remains *elevated*. It is not yet fully under control. But it's sufficiently low that I can now be transported to an open bed at EH.

# Part 2

# Recovery Begins
## Emory Hospital

I failed to save my grandma from death. Like so many living in poverty, preventable circumstances killed her. My mother, although considered middle class, met similar conditions: diabetes, hypertension, stroke, hemorrhage, abrasions, wounds and their infection. My savings were depleted. Credit cards, maxed. I began throwing collection letters from hospitals into the trash. I stopped answering my phone to avoid speaking to debt agencies . . . I could no longer afford to keep my mother alive.— Donald Edem Quist, *To Those Bounded*

And yet, it is to my mother—and all of our mothers who were not famous—that I went in search of the secret of what has fed that muzzled and often mutilated, but vibrant, creative spirit that the black woman has inherited, and that pops out in wild and unlikely places to this day.—Alice Walker, *In Search of Our Mothers' Gardens*

15

# Somebody Prayed for Me

ALL KNOWING—AND ALL KNOWLEDGE—IS contextual. Knowing is seldom, if ever, devoid of uncertainty because our knowing, as human beings, is never complete or absolute. In the coming weeks and months, I hold in tension knowing and uncertainty—knowing what is required for my recovery and uncertainty about my ability to prevent future strokes. Having a stroke increases my risk for stroke. I must hold the two together peacefully in my body. I cannot, will not, live in fear or anxiety; it will not help my cause. But for the first few months after my stroke, my greatest fear is that I might suffer another stroke.

Similarly, I encourage my students to embrace the tension between our "knowing" what a text means *and* the vulnerable uncertainty of remaining open to the possibility that our "knowing" is partial, possibly incorrect, troublesome, and even harmful to ourselves and others. Be confident and humble. Be open to knowing differently and holding various and even opposing (or seemingly opposing) ideas, practices, and other knowledge production in conversation without being dismissive of or demonizing others.

I know that many people are praying for me from the moment that they learn that I've had a stroke. I certainly believe in the power of prayer. I pray even when I'm unsure about how God works or if God cares; it's a lifelong habit I cannot shake. I pray, seldom on my knees; prayer is prayer. As small children, my mother made us pray, taught us to pray, showed us what praying looks like. We couldn't eat without repeating the words "Bless this food we are about to receive for the nourishment of our bodies. Amen."

We couldn't go to bed without saying "Now I lay me down to sleep. I pray the Lord my soul to keep. If I should die before I wake, I pray the Lord my soul to take. Amen." My mother, like many Black Christian mothers (and other mothers), prayed in the King's English: "Thou art good to us, O God." The King James Version of the Bible (KJV) is what she knew best and most when it came to Scripture and the language of faith. She recited Scripture from the KJV. That's all many Christians know. The King's English is God's language for many folks.

After my mother became unable to walk and in her later years, she'd sit on the side of her bed and rock her body back and forth, rubbing her knees. I found myself doing the same thing whenever I was in pain. It became an instinctive habit so that, even after the pain left, I'd rock back and forth, rubbing both hands on my knees in tandem. On the nights that my mother sat up rocking on the side of her bed, one of us children would help her back into the bed.

"Mommy, are you in pain at night when you sit on the side of your bed? What are you thinking about?" I'd ask.

"I'm praying for my children," she softly replied.

There's a "negro spiritual" that goes like this: "Somebody prayed for me, had me on their mind and prayed for me . . . my mother prayed for me . . . my sister prayed for me . . . my brother prayed for me . . . had me on their mind."[1] My mother is long gone. I've felt "orphaned" since she died in March 2009. But I know my sisters are praying for me. If my brother Fred were alive, he'd be praying for me too. I know that my peer mentoring sister-friends, Drs. Sheila Winborne and Janice Farrell, are praying for me. Dr. Angela Sims continually prays for me and sends gifts. I know that my long-time friend Sharon Ozonuwe who calls, and visits from New Jersey, is praying for me. Somebody somewhere is praying for me. I'm praying too.

My theology, my human-constructed God talk, has changed over the years. I imagine and hope that it will continue to change or evolve as long as I'm willing to hold in tension the inscrutability or mystery of God and the limits of my fallible humanity. I never believed nor was I taught to believe, at least not by my mother, that God cares more about Christians than other folks. I don't believe God *favors* Christians over other folks. I don't believe that tithing is a down payment or a layaway plan for purchasing the special miracles and blessings of God.

---

1. "Somebody Prayed for Me" was written by Dorothy Norwood and Alvin Darling in 1935.

When did faith in God become knowing exactly what God will do, how she will act, and for whom? For me, where I stand spiritually today, faith is an exercise in and the practice of hope. I hold uncertainty, hope, fear, and faith in the same body. My truth is I'm scared. Not all the time. But I have my moments, hours, and days. I don't know what the future looks like. Who does? A life-threatening illness forces you to live a minute, hour, and day at a time. The threat hovers over my life, until it doesn't. It's bigger than me and anything or anyone I know. So I pray. And I'm glad somebody else is praying for me.

## 16

# Blood, Sodium, and Water

At EH I have a small private room with a bathroom that I'm never physically able to use. It is at EH that I discover I cannot walk. Due to the effects of the stroke, the dying brain cells continued to weaken and damage the connection between my brain and the rest of my body while I was in the ICU.

I don't recall the doctors or nurses wearing face masks. They may have done so, but I don't recall. Most doctors who visit me stand at the foot of my bed spouting information at me. Only one doctor stands within five to six feet of me. The only woman doctor who visits several times positions herself in closer proximity to me on the right-hand side of my bed. I don't remember one doctor at Emory Hospital touching my body.

I soon learn from the kidney doctor as he stands at the foot of my bed that I have been "drinking too much water" and "washing the sodium from [my] body." My sodium levels are too low. I think, *I can't win*. In early May, my primary care doctor asked me if I was drinking enough water. I assured her that I drink lots of water. I don't think she believed me. I have suffered from dry mouth for several years now. I assume it is the result of menopause, having received no definitive explanation from any health care or dental worker. I can't ever drink enough water; I drink water while eating (never did most of my life) to aid in digestion and between meals when talking a lot. Over-the-counter remedies don't work well or long term. Biotene gel provides temporary relief and helps when placed in my mouth before I lecture. For the entire duration of my relatively short stay at EH, the nurses administer sodium pills to me and limit my liquid intake.

    The people who touch me most often, pricking my skin and breaking my flesh, are the phlebotomists who draw my blood four times each day, including at 4:00 AM. They are watching my sodium levels. I cannot stand the sight of my own blood being drained from my body. I am grateful when skilled phlebotomists and nurses inflict as little pain as possible. Once my sister Sina refused to let a nurse attempt to put a needle in my mother's arm a third time: "Naw! You need to go get somebody else who's more skilled or knows what they're doing," she demanded. Sina doesn't mince her words. She don't play! Sina trained and worked as a phlebotomist for the Red Cross for a brief stint. I don't remember why she quit.

## 17

# Can't Feed Myself!

I CANNOT FEED MYSELF, which is quite inconvenient now that I'm allowed to eat solid foods. Both my left and right arms and hands are quite weak, but the right side is weaker. So much for being right-handed. The fingers on my right hand are numb and not functioning properly. Normal dexterity is gone. I depend on the nurses—overworked nurses responsible for too many patients—to feed me. I cannot open the containers of Jell-O, applesauce, juice, or milk. I cannot tear open the packets of salt, sugar, and condiments. I cannot remove the paper from my straws. I cannot even hold my eating utensils and don't have the strength to pick up a small glass of juice or water.

The solid food served at EH is a tremendous improvement over the liquid and soft, tasteless food the nurses rounded up for me in the ICU. My stomach is much smaller now. I cannot eat much food; it will be some time before my body accepts normal-sized meals. But EH serves some of the best watermelon I've enjoyed anywhere.

I am frightened at how helpless I am. I'm dependent on the nurses and my two constant visitors, Lisa Weaver and Christine Yoder, to help me. It's daunting. It's scary. But I'm alive and I'm fighting to recover my life.

# 18

# Day Two
## Angels

ON MY FIRST DAY in EH, my nurse, a middle-aged Black woman, cares for me very well. She skillfully and gently gives me a much-needed bed bath, pouring warm soapy water over my parched body from head to toe. We talk as she bathes me. "I treat people the way I would want to be treated," she insists. My body is grateful; I am refreshed! My nurse changes my bedding and continues holding friendly conversation with me as she feeds me my breakfast and lunch. All this wonderful and necessary care is short-lived.

On my second day in EH, my nurse arrives complaining that her back hurts as she sits to open the various cartons and packages of food on the breakfast tray that has been left for me. I feel badly that she is suffering and yet has to do the work expected of her as a nurse for the next eight hours. I also wonder why she is unloading her pain on me, her patient who still needs her assistance and care. I discover during my stay at the hospital (and later at the rehabilitation hospital) that too many nurses are themselves physically unhealthy in ways that interfere with them performing their jobs well. Some are merely trying to hold out until they can retire. Others are fed up with unhelpful and oppressive institutional systems and structures. Some are incompetent and surly. But they are all stretched thin. All of this impacts patient care and recovery.

In the Bible, angels visit warriors and prep them for the battlefields where tribes, peoples, and kingdoms go to war. An angel of Yahweh appears to Gideon, who is hiding from the Midianites in the winepress, and declares to him that he is a mighty warrior even as he stands body-deep in fear. An angel of Yahweh visits the young Egyptian slave woman named Hagar in the wilderness as she struggles to decide her next move after fleeing her enslaver Sarah's wrath (Gen 16). At this point, Hagar is pregnant following the rape orchestrated by Sarah and perpetrated by Sarah's aged but fertile husband, Abraham. The angel sends Hagar back into the war zone, namely Sarah and Abraham's house, with a promise that she will bear a son and of a better fertile future. In the Acts of the Apostles, angels visit the cells of incarcerated men like the apostles Peter, John, Saul (aka Paul), and Silas. These men are part of an internal Jewish conflict over the content and impact of the apostles' preaching and activities, which also draws the attention of the Roman authorities. There are no stories of angels visiting the women and men of the Way whom Saul/Paul persecutes and incarcerates prior to his call to join them.

The angel Gabriel visits both Mary and Zechariah, Elizabeth's husband, to deliver the news of the women's precarious, untimely, unexpected, and unconventional (to say the least) pregnancies at which they are compelled to rejoice; it's God's favor. There is no angelic visitation for Elizabeth; she only learns she is pregnant as her stomach swells. Narratives like these unrealistically omit the trauma that childbirth inflicts upon a woman's body under normal circumstances, let alone under unusual, even troublesome and warlike, circumstances. I imagine that both women bear and fend off all kinds of assaults and insults due to the suspicious circumstances of their pregnancies. So angels are not simply angelic (i.e., kind, gentle, pure, innocent, heavenly/otherworldly) in their demeanor or in terms of the content and impact of the message they bear or the very worldly events, and consequences of those events, their words set in motion. Interestingly, they are all men; all the angels are men. When named, they are given male names.

But I don't believe all angels are men, even if we find none with traditional female names in the Bible. All of my doctors and nurses—the compassionate, competent, complicated, helpful, harsh, hurtful, and horrible ones—are angels. Angels are not God, which makes them as imperfect and vulnerable as other created beings. They are commissioned to assist me and other patients as we recover.

My nurse is angelic, in a refreshingly therapeutic way, on my first day at EH. It turns out that day one is the exception and not the rule. Bed baths and the changing of my bedding are supposed to be daily routines. I never again experience a bed bath like the one my nurse treated me to that first day. And other necessities, like changing my bedding, are hit and miss.

# 19

# God Didn't Cause Me to Have a Stroke

A SIXTY-TWO-YEAR-OLD BLACK CHRISTIAN woman with a Caribbean accent comes into my room to draw my blood. Out of the blue, she testifies, as I lay in my bed unable to walk, "I am blessed. I am sixty-two years old and have never been seriously ill or hospitalized." I feel assaulted by her shot of religious superiority. After a brief pause, I counter, "Well, I am sixty-five and a half years old. And this is my first hospitalization and incidence of a serious debilitating illness." In other words, live a little longer and you might not be so lucky, blessed, or however you choose to name it.

Stroke survivors and other seriously ill people are not people whom God chose not to bless. I don't believe that God's grace, gifts, or favor are reserved for people who wear their spirituality or religion on their tongues, belong to a certain denomination or religion, or use all the acceptable or approved religious jargon when they speak. Stroke survivors and other seriously ill persons do not need callous, harmful theologies or ideologies flung at them, especially not from health care providers. Miss me with that nonsense.

Recently, the actor, singer, and comedian Jamie Foxx released a Netflix special in which he testifies that he suffered a stroke.[1] He shares how it debilitated him and how he struggled to recover. He, like anyone who suffers a serious, life-threatening, devastating illness, wanted to know "why

1. Foxx and Hamilton, *Jamie Foxx*.

me?" "Why now?" Foxx's sister is deeply religious. According to him, she prayed on her knees just outside the operating room as he underwent brain surgery. Perhaps she influenced or helped him find answers to his questions—answers that he needed to find peace, to make sense of what had happened to him, and to make peace with the disruption in his life and the damage to his body. In his Netflix special, Foxx shares his conclusion with an audience that responds with "amens," "hallelujahs," and shouts, just like a congregation in a traditional Black church on Sunday morning. Foxx testifies that God caused him to have a stroke because he had not been to church in a long time. I don't want to begrudge Foxx what he chooses and needs to believe, but God didn't bless me with a stroke. Life exacts its pound of flesh, and none of us is exempt. Oppressive polices, practices, and ideologies cause and/or exacerbate illness.

It is human to ask, "Why me?" or "Where is God in all this?" Marcellus Robinson, my former pastor of the Bladensburg Seventh-day Adventist Church in Bladensburg, Maryland, where I once served, asked in a sermon, "If not you, then who?" Who should suffer a stroke instead of me? Black communities have a 50 percent higher risk of stroke than white people and other racial and ethnicity groups. Black men are 70 percent more likely to die of stroke than white men.[2] Chances are that I or somebody I love or know will suffer a stroke. According to the American Heart Association, "Black women are more likely to die from stroke" than all other groups.[3] An answer to "Why me?" is *Because of racism, sexism, classism, misogynoir, and poverty. And of course, all these are connected to the insatiable lust for unregulated capitalism.*

---

2. Office of Minority Health, "Stroke and African Americans."
3. American Heart Association, "Facts, Causes and Risks of Stroke."

## 20

# Day Three
## Retaliation

ON MY THIRD DAY in EH, Lisa Weaver visits me. She is sitting in the chair in my room chatting with me when the male charge nurse, a middle-aged Black man, pops in and dutifully asks, "How are we treating you, Ms. Smith?" Glancing at Lisa, with whom I already discussed the lack of consistency in my treatment and care, I hesitantly ask, "Is it hospital practice to change the bedding and to give patients bed baths every day?" After day one, my nurse changes only the disposable white and blue pad placed under my body and not all of my bedding. I already know what the charge nurse's response should be, but a small part of me wonders if perhaps hospital policy has changed during and after the COVID crisis (as it has in some hotels, which now only change linen for longer stays or if guests request the service). The charge nurse responds, "Yes, it is our practice to bathe patients and change bedding daily. Why? Is this not happening?" "It is not," I answer. I then express concern about how he will address the problem. I want to avoid retaliation from my nurses. The charge nurse assures me that he will be very tactful in addressing the issue. But something goes wrong.

The next morning, the nurse who had given me the glorious therapeutic bed bath and cordially talked with me while feeding me, all the while boasting, "I treat people the way I would want to be treated," assumes a distant, frigid posture with few words to spare. Her demeanor and treatment of me changes drastically and abruptly. Bear in mind that, at this point, I have not yet received any occupational therapy (and wouldn't until I am admitted to the rehab hospital). Occupational therapy equips patients to overcome physical, emotional, and social challenges that interfere with the performance of daily tasks like bathing, clothing, and feeding themselves. But my nurse now callously insists that I feed myself, as she stands behind me with her arms folded, looking over my shoulder while I struggle to do what I cannot yet remember how to do and do not have the strength and dexterity to perform. I do not break down, but I am deeply hurt. I am helpless, but she refuses to help me. But I will not let her win. I struggle, with little success. The nurse gives an inch and reaches over to open the food packages for me, but that is it. Our conversations over meals cease. She has tossed her moral-ethical compass to the wind when she learns that I expected the care that all patients deserve and need.

I don't imagine I am the only patient in the hospital suffering from such neglect. The man whose yells drift into the hallway around mealtime and other times may be one of those patients. When I told the charge nurse about not receiving a daily bed bath and not having my bedding changed, I hadn't mentioned the nurse's name. But she obviously knows I complained. She took it personally; I become her nemesis rather than a stroke patient needing her care and for whom she is paid to care. I'm grateful on the days that she is assigned to another patient and not to me.

## 21

# Left Alone

THAT EXPERIENCE OF NEGLECT is not my last while in EH. The next one is almost a nightmare. It occurs late at night. A younger African American nurse working the night shift divides her time between me, other patients, and apparently the break room. I cannot walk eight to ten feet to the bathroom in my room. Nor can I manage a few steps without assistance. The nurse helps me ambulate from my bed to the portable toilet seat that sits against the wall about two or three feet from my bed. The hospital advises me and other stroke patients to never leave (or return to) our hospital beds without calling for assistance. Understandably, the hospital doesn't want anyone falling and injuring themselves. Well, the nurse never returns to help me back into my bed. After searching for the gray cord attached to the call button, I see that it is entangled in the bed railing. I cannot untangle it. I cannot reach the call button. I wait a long time, perhaps an hour or so, but my nurse doesn't return, and nobody else comes by my room. I think to myself, *I am not sitting on this toilet all night*. So I decide that I must try to get into the bed since nobody is coming to help me. I manage to stand to my feet. Almost like a four-foot, eleven-inch ping pong ball, I stumble a few steps forward and bang my left side into the rolling cart that is positioned three to four feet from my bed. Barely skipping a beat, I bounce off the cart like an eight-ball shot off the side of a pool table and fall onto the bed. I feel bruised, accomplished, and relieved when I hit the soft bed. Inching and scooting my body toward the middle of the bed, I thank God. After my breathing slows and I'm calm, I fall off to sleep. The phlebotomist arrives at

4:00 AM to draw my blood. Looking back; it's quite funny. But at the time, I feel hurt, scared, and abandoned.

At about 8:00 AM, I inform the charge nurse that I was left to stay on the portable toilet all night, that the nurse never returned, that nobody came by, that I could not get to the call button, and that I stumbled back into the bed.

"Did you hit floor or not?"

"No, I didn't hit the floor. But I fell into the cart and bruised my body."

He's not concerned.

## 22

# Another Angel

ONE AFTERNOON A LATINA woman enters my room, dusts the surfaces here and there, and empties the trash. She speaks Spanish *y un poco* (and a little) English as she moves about the room to my left. She picks up the green flowering plant that is hidden among other things cluttering the windowsill and places it where I can enjoy it in all of its beauty. My younger sister Lenora sent me the plant. "It's too beautiful to sit in the corner; you can enjoy it better here," she says. "Muchas gracias," I respond.

Her thoughtful gesture means so much to me. She asks if she can offer a prayer for me. I recognize the Spanish word for prayer (*oración*) from my Spanish language studies. When I lived in Detroit, I learned some Spanish with a small group led by a native speaker from Spain. I continued my studies using the Duolingo app. I can read more Spanish than I can speak. According to the app, I am 40 percent fluent in Spanish. I respectfully disagree. Duolingo is far too forgiving and gracious. But it doesn't matter to me that I can't understand every word the woman says to me. She demonstrates her kindness. I sense her compassion. After praying for me, the young woman leaves the room, having uplifted my spirit. In difficult situations, kind gestures like hers are life-giving. When remembered, they help us to remain hopeful and resilient in the face of neglect and hurt.

The Latina woman returns at about three that afternoon. She pokes her head into the doorway to say goodbye and that she will pray for my recovery. I had never seen that young woman before she entered my room that day, and I never see her again. She was an angel.

## Another Angel

My mother shared stories of her encounters with angels. I recall one particular story better than the others. She had been invited to a house party on the south side of Columbus, Ohio. My mother rode the public bus to the south side. When she stepped off the bus, a man approached her. "You don't want to go to that house," he said. Instead of going to the party, she waited for the next bus going back home. God, my mother believed, had dispatched an angel to warn her of the danger awaiting her at that house party. The next day the local news reported that somebody committed murder in that very house on that same night.

## 23

# Physical Therapy Begins

My stay at EH lasts less than a week, but they waste no time dispatching a physical therapist to my room to help get me on my feet and walking. Early in my stay, a slim African American woman, Tynisha, arrives in my room to introduce herself as the physical therapist assigned to me. She returns the next day with a walker, expecting or insisting that I stand up. I don't want to stand up because my entire body is so weak. I have lost so much muscle strength that I don't recognize my body.

"Scoot over near the edge of bed," Tynisha instructs. "Move your left leg over the side of the bed. Now move your right leg over the side. Now, use your arms to push yourself up to a seated position on the side of the bed." She is standing on the left side of the bed in front of me the entire time, helping me with each move. Just sitting up, even with Tynisha's help, is a great accomplishment. But we are not finished yet.

Next, while I'm seated on the side of the bed, Tynisha places the walker in front of me and places my hands on it. She positions her arms under my armpits and lifts me to my feet. Propped up by the walker and Tynisha's arms, I linger on my feet for a few seconds. Then I plop back down onto the bed. I'm exhausted and smiling because of what we've achieved.

The next day, Tynisha insists that I walk from my bed to the bathroom door with the walker. Again, the most difficult thing to do is just getting out of the bed. "I don't feel like standing up today." Tynisha cuts her eyes at me as if to say, "I didn't come here for you to do nothing. You can get up. I'll wait." Like an intimidated army recruit, I get up, and I try to perform exactly as she expects. With her assistance, we follow the same routine as yesterday for sitting on the side of the bed and standing up on the walker. I don't do it alone. When Tynisha challenges my body, the connection between my body and brain is being rebuilt little by little. I'm so proud of myself after each of our brief sessions together. Getting started is always the most difficult part. In less than a week, we advance from a slow sluggish walk from the left side of the bed to the bathroom door, to sitting on the toilet, standing up off the toilet, and walking back to the bed with the walker.

At our last session, Tynisha announces, "We are going to walk in the hallway today."

I protest, "Not the hallway. It's too long."

"We won't go far," she assures me.

Tynisha is still asking me to do things that my body finds very difficult, painful, and even foreign, even with the walker. But she isn't taking "no" for an answer. We follow the routine for getting me on my feet with the walker. We, the walker and me, make it into the hallway, which is about the same distance as the walk from my bed to the bathroom. My struggle is now exposed to the rest of the world, the world outside my hospital room. Before now, I have not encountered or interacted with any other patients. The change of scenery from staring at four walls to a peek into the rooms of other patients lying in their beds makes me feel less lonely and separate from the rest of the world. The hallway traffic is minimal. It surprises me to find so few people milling around; it shouldn't have. After all, many patients are in the same shape as me, unable to move their bodies or leave their beds except by wheelchair or walker. They, like me, rely on health care workers to feed, bathe, and change them—health care workers who are overworked, tired, unwell, cranky, and/or fed up with institutional bureaucracy.

Tynisha keeps her word. We don't go far before turning back. Leaning on the walker and flanked by my physical therapist, I slowly and deliberately place one foot in front of the other until I reach the threshold of my room. That was my last physical therapy session with her before being transferred to Emory Rehab Hospital (ERH). According to Tynisha's May 30, 2023 notes in MyChart, my strengths are "ability to acquire knowledge, insight into problems, attitude, premorbid level of function." She assesses me as having "decreased strength, decreased endurance, impaired balance, decreased mobility, gait instability, fall risk, impaired transfers, needs patient/family/caregiver education, needs discharge planning," but my prognosis and rehab potential are "good."

## 24

# Outside World

OTHER THAN LISA WEAVER, Christine Yoder, Marcia Riggs, and the health care workers, I do not let the outside world into my hospital room. I have no interest in watching the television; it is never turned on. Before my stroke, my psychotherapist Renee warned, "You might be on the verge of burnout." I was doing what was expected of me as a professor and an academic. But I *desired* to do very little; I performed. So I planned a vacation in January 2023 to Cancun, which used to be one of my favorite vacation destinations. Renee challenged me not to pack a single book, not even a novel, for my trip. I thought to myself, *Oh, please, it won't hurt to take a novel; I haven't read a novel in awhile.* I had so many on my bookshelf that I'd love to read. So I failed the challenge and carried one novel with me to Cancun. I cannot recall which novel. I couldn't bring myself to read it while on vacation. I couldn't even open it.

Looking back, I believe that I suffered from post-traumatic stress from watching the unrelenting barrage of videos featuring police officers shooting Black people in their backs as they ran away or sat in their homes, or snuffing the life from their bodies by pressing knees into their necks or their backs while their hands were cuffed behind them, chests and noses pushed into cemented and paved roads. Black people were and continue to be killed in police custody and in jails. Those videos on replay and the incessant analysis and chatter about them on MSNBC stressed and traumatized me. All the videos and noise of domestic and state-sanctioned violence against Black bodies made me ill, and I felt helpless. But I, and many others, would not allow Tamir Rice, Michael Brown, George Floyd, Breonna Taylor, Sandra Bland, and so many more to die in relative silence without protest and outrage, without at least saying their names. I posted on Facebook, Twitter, and Instagram, and I wrote about their deaths in my writings and in short blog posts on my website.

Every Saturday, I typically rest. I don't do any academic work or housework beyond preparing my own meals, but I don't wash dishes. On Saturdays, I am a total slouch. I convinced myself that Saturdays off the grid, in addition to healthy eating and exercise, was enough reprieve to stave off burnout or exhaustion. But before I had my stroke, the thing I did not stop doing on Saturdays was watching cable news. So it makes sense that I never once turn on the TV during my hospitalization, nor do I desire to read a book, fiction or nonfiction.

## 25

# Ready for Rehab

A SOCIAL WORKER VISITS me to ask where I would like to go for rehabilitation. Evidently, I've made enough progress during the short stay at EH to move to the next stage of my stroke recovery journey, which may also mean that my insurance insists upon it. "I'll return in a day or so to give you time to think about where you'd like to go," she says. I've never been here before, in this post-stroke body or in a hospital recovering from a serious illness. I have no idea how to choose a rehabilitation facility. I don't know any close family members who have been in one. I know no one who has been in one here in Georgia. When the social worker returns, she asks, "Would you like to go to Emory Rehab Hospital or another rehabilitation facility?" Emory's brand is familiar to me now, and time is of the essence. It's not like I have the emotional, mental, or physical bandwidth to research rehabs near me or in Georgia. I elect to go to ERH. May 31, 2024, is my last day at EH.

# Part 3

# Fighting My Way Back
## Emory Rehabilitation Hospital

*As a trained neuroanatomist, I believed in the plasticity of my brain—its agility to repair, replace, and retrain its neutral circuitry.—Jill Bolte Taylor, PhD,* My Stroke of Insight: A Brain Scientist's Personal Journey

26

# Arrival

The mobile bed ride from EH to ERH is precarious. It's just me and the driver. No other hallway traffic. It's the longest ride I've taken since being ill and hospitalized. It's tortuous. A significant stretch of the journey is like a roller-coaster ride, descending and ascending hills and negotiating curves in the long tunnel that stretches for part of the route. A little spooked and nervous midway a descent, I look down and notice I'm not strapped into the bed. Fudgesicle! I think about shouting at the driver, "Hey, stop. My seat belt is not buckled!" But I don't. A sudden stop might cause us to roll forwards. I become the back-seat driver my older sister hates. Difference is, I cannot press the imaginary brake with my numb, stiff feet. Sina hates it when I press those brakes. At the speed at which we are traveling, I pray we, the driver and me, reach our destination soon and without incident. Eventually, we reach flat ground and brighter light. Shish! Thank God!

On May 31, 2023, I arrive at ERH. What we know about grocery store chains, food franchises, and name brand services and products is the same for hospitals. Two entities or hospitals—Emory Hospital and Emory Rehab—can carry the same brand name but provide unique experiences that are better, worse, similar, different, or consistently the same. It is like how the numerous departments, schools, or colleges in a university system—law school, college of medicine, school of theology, and so on—are not all equal, nor are they consistently excellent, mediocre, or horrible across the system. Significant distinguishing factors in hospital systems are the doctors, other health care workers, and food. No doubt EH has a better chef than ERH. Both have excellent, mediocre, indifferent, and cruel health care workers. Hospitals have their alter egos that differ from their general public image, and they also have their scales of care that range from compassionate and extremely competent to negligent and scandalously harmful.

It's late in the evening when I arrive and well past dinner time, as I remember. EH couldn't transport me before a bed became available. I am not checked into ERH until the next day because the system is closed, as I understand it. Arriving in the middle of the week also puts me at a disadvantage food-wise. On Fridays, patients select their food choices from the menu options for the following week. So I must wait a couple days to select my meal preferences for next week. In the meantime, I'm served whatever is available. Soon I discover the precarity of my predicament because very few menu items are eatable. Before the stroke, I was neither overweight (maybe slightly) nor my ideal weight. The women in my family carry their weight primarily in their hips. I went from about 132 pounds pre-stroke (I'm only 4'11") to about a hundred pounds or slightly under in a relatively short period of about twenty-five days during May. To ensure I don't dwindle away, I ask a nurse assistant, "Is there any chance I can get some Ensure, chocolate?" "Certainly, I'll look in the fridge to see if I can locate some for you, Ms. Smith." She returns with several bottles of chocolate Ensure. "Thank you so much!" These bottles will hold me until next week.

## 27

# Dr. Justin and the Quiz

On Wednesday, May 31, 2023, the same day I arrive at ERH, I meet Dr. Justin (his first name, apparently his preference for addressing him). He is a tall thirty- or fortysomething, white-haired white man. Dr. Justin is the senior resident doctor, I believe. I don't recall ever telling Dr. Justin that I have an earned PhD, but he knows. Perhaps he asked me at some point, and I forgot that conversation, or he read it in my patient history.

"Dr. Smith, do you know why I'm wearing a mask?" Dr. Justin asks.

"Yes, to protect me."

"That's right, to protect you and to protect us," he replies.

"Do you know why you are here? Do you know where you are? Do you know what month it is? The day of the week? Your full name? The month, day and year of your birth?"

I ace the quiz.

The entire sixteen days I spend at ERH, all my doctors, nurse assistants, nurses, and therapists wear masks. I only ever see two or three of my physical therapists without a mask and only briefly when we go outdoors or are in a closed office where there are only the two of us present. I wouldn't recognize them on the street if I saw them. In some cases, that's a good thing, but in others, it saddens me, because should I run into any of them in public, I won't be able to tell them how much their care meant to me.

# 28

# (Dis)Respect, Patient Preference, and Gender

As I am a new patient, the first nurse assigned to me must perform a wound assessment, checking my body from head to toe for bruises, lacerations, or wounds of any kind. My nurse is a man of African descent, originally from Kenya, I later discover.

"Ms. Smith, my name is Paul [not his actual name], your nurse. I must check your body for wounds."

"I prefer that a woman nurse assesses my body," I respond.

He acts offended—as if my request is a personal assault on him—and attempts to ignore my request. I persist. He summons his nurse assistant, a Black woman, who positions herself on my right side near the bottom of the bed and starts to uncover me from the bottom up. Paul doesn't leave the room but stands at the foot of the bed, his head and eyes following the movement of the bedding upward. His intention is to check my body with the nurse assistant, despite my preference. The nurse assistant halts when I raise my voice. "I said I want a woman to assess my body!" A resentful Paul finally leaves the room. I'm disturbed and angered that he disrespects me by attempting to ignore my personal preference, as if it doesn't matter what I want. As if I'm being silly and unreasonable. His behavior is creepy. I'm also angry because patients who can't advocate for themselves are at the mercy of health care workers like Paul who don't respect patients' preferences and bodies—at least not women's, it seems.

In fewer than ten minutes, the woman nurse assistant assesses my body and notes that I have no wounds. Paul returns after she notifies him of the results.

That isn't my last troubling encounter with Paul. He serves as my nurse several other days.

On another day he asks, "Don't you like male nurses? I know you don't like me."

"I never said I don't like you! I don't know you."

He is gaslighting me, attempting to blame me for his own insecurities and his lack of respect for my wishes as a woman patient. But it won't work.

The only other male nurse that I encounter at ERH is Sam (not his real name), a trainee; he is a pleasant, tall, slim young white man. Keisha, one of the most capable, caring, and efficient nurses assigned to me at ERH, is training Sam. Keisha is a thirtyish, pleasant and attractive African American woman. Actually, she is a nurse assistant; in my mind she is a nurse! Ms. Brown (my first roommate) and I love Keisha! And Keisha loves us.

Sam pops into my room. "Ms. Smith, I'm Sam. Keisha said you need help using the bed pan."

"Hi Sam, please don't take this the wrong way, but I prefer that a woman assists me."

Sam's response is nothing like Paul's. Without hesitation, he replies, "It's no problem, Ms. Smith. I understand perfectly. No need to explain."

He gets it! He's been raised and trained well!

# 29

# Dr. Milton and Still Me

I MEET DR. MILTON, the attending physician, on Thursday morning, June 1, when he, Dr. Justin, and a junior resident (who never says a mumbalin' word) make their rounds. Dr. Justin, positioned at the foot of my bed, introduces Dr. Milton to me.

"This is Dr. Smith," Dr. Justin says.

"What kind of doctor? . . . DEd, MD, PhD . . . ?" Dr. Milton asks, standing on the right side of my bed with one foot forward.

"PhD."

"Retired?"

"No."

Dr. Milton joins Dr. Justin at the foot of my hospital bed where they discuss the numbness in my feet. I'm listening like I'm the "fly on the wall," but of course, I'm not. I'm the wide-awake woman in the bed. Dr. Milton decides to test the feeling in my big toes. Starting with my right foot, he yanks up the blanket and sheet, which are tucked securely under the mattress, and exposes my feet.

"Close your eyes and tell me if I'm moving your toe up or down," Dr. Milton instructs.

"Up . . . down . . . up . . . up . . . down," I say, as he bends my right toe backward and forward.

Dr. Milton switches to the big toe on my left foot.

"Up . . . up . . . uh down . . . uh up . . . down," I speculate.

"Now you're guessing."

Eyes still closed, a burst of laughter escapes from my gut, shattering what should be a sobering moment. Not sure why, but I'm not terrified by the possibility that my feet might have some paralysis. Maybe it's because the numbness doesn't prevent me from standing on my feet. My knee-jerk reaction is a sign that I'm still me. As an afterthought, I should have said to Dr. Milton, "You gave me only two choices. You didn't say 'Up, down, or I don't know.' So I guessed." That's the detail-oriented me.

Much of my life, I've found humor in situations that others don't find funny or not as funny. Because of comments made to me about my laughter, a younger me learned to stifle it. As I get older, I'm less concerned with what other people think. If a younger me was in church and the preacher said something or someone did something I found funny, a surge of laughter would slice the air before I could suppress it. I admit, sometimes it happened at a most inconvenient or inappropriate time; but it was never planned. Many years ago, I sang in the chorus (my first and last) that was organized for usher's day at the Hilltop Seventh-day Adventist Church in Columbus, Ohio, my home church at the time. I was the youngest member of the chorus and one of several in the small group who couldn't hold a tune. My mother was trained in classical music as a vocalist and pianist from about eight years old through high school. She once said she had an opportunity to travel with the Louis Armstrong band, but she couldn't see herself as a young woman traveling with a group of men. Mommy tried to teach me to sing and play the piano, but she decided I was too tone deaf. I can't remember the song we were singing for usher's day; but when we started singing the second stanza, the director, standing directly in front of me, sang the wrong stanza, the third one. Worse, her voice rang out above ours, out of tune and off script. I managed to stifle the sound of my laughter, but like a caged bird, the sound I tried to muffle would not be absolutely contained. The laughter, shut up in my belly, shook my body. I stopped singing; my face turned red. When the leader nudged me with her elbow, I nearly burst. Laughter is contagious; I didn't mean for it to be, not on that day at that moment. Soon, other chorus members were laughing as silently as they could. This church was not your traditional Black church. You could hear a pin drop during worship. An "amen" would seldom break the silence. To many, I was just being Mitzi.

I love to laugh. My mother loved to laugh and would crack herself up telling a funny story. Her laughter was contagious. Before she reached the end of the story, we'd all be triggered by her laughter, laughing until our bodies shook and tears ran down our cheeks. She told us about the time she was angry with our dad. Somebody told her he was down at the corner bar, drinking away food or rent money. After serving in World War II, he couldn't stop drinking. Mom flew down to the bar. He was in the bathroom. Didn't stop her. She confronted him while he was sitting on the toilet. Evidently, she took a bottle with her into the men's restroom, located the stall he was in, and cracked him over the head with the bottle. He burst out laughing! My mother laughed hysterically every time she told the story. My father wasn't hurt. He was too numbed up by the alcohol.

Laughter and music, all kinds of upbeat music, are my energy drink. I love inspirational music, Black gospel, seventies, eighties, and nineties Motown or soul, a little bit of country, reggae. I'm less likely to sit too long under the spell of writing if I'm listening to Tina, Beyoncé, Luther, Mickey Guyton, Jon Batiste, Tupac, MJ, Janet, Patti, and others. They pull me to my feet; they are irresistible dance partners. Music is more effective than setting the alarm on my iPhone; the sound of the alarm is mostly annoying. When I remember to set it, I tend to ignore it until it shuts itself off. Ironically, the music doesn't distract me. Music and laughter are two loves that lift my spirit when I'm down, if I remember to reach for them. I love a hilarious comedy or comedian. I love the comedy of Robin Williams and Bernie Mack. Lucille Ball is too outrageously silly to be funny, but Carol Burnett easily makes me laugh. I love Wanda Sykes's comedy. I recently discovered Josh Johnson, a young African American stand-up comedian whose routines are full of critical social commentary. In a recent YouTube show, Josh said,

> I don't know if ya'll saw what's happening in LA. But the archdiocese in LA just settled for $750 million dollars with the lawsuits of everyone who had claimed abuse while they were patrons of the church . . . That brings the Catholic Church's total payout to $1.5 Billion . . . Anyone else would be closed . . . There's no other company I could really think of that could do that much harm and be able to afford the payout. You'd have to be a gun manufacturer or something . . . It feels less like justice because they had it [the money to pay], just laying around. You gotta make them pay a number that they genuinely don't know. "Oh, that I don't know if we could do." That's exactly how much I want . . . How can that not affect your faith? This is supposed to be a place where you can lay down every burden, not pick up extra.[1]

1. Johnson, "Almighty Payout."

# 30

# Rhythm and Rhyme of Therapy

At ERH, Monday through Friday for about three to four hours a day, I am scheduled for occupational, physical, and speech therapy. The day begins at 6:30 or 7:00 am. The first week is most challenging, particularly with physical and occupational therapy. I have little muscle strength. I tire easily. My body craves sleep and rest. Part of me is excited to get started with therapy, considering the progress I made with the physical therapist at EH. At ERH, instead of one therapist who spends ten or fifteen minutes with me (that's all I could handle at that stage of my stroke), three to four therapists arrive almost in succession each day to collect me in my wheelchair for forty-five-minute sessions. Part of my body wants to say, "Slow your roll. Not so fast." Another part of me thinks, "Let's get this show on the road." Sometimes my body is dragged along kicking and screaming by the rigorous, structured therapy schedule and excellent committed therapists who show up in my room.

For the first few days to a week, I'm less than enamored with the compulsory torturous sessions. As my body responds, my attitude changes. As my attitude shifts, my body becomes more amenable to the positive change I struggle for. By the beginning of week two, I'm silently complaining about the lack of therapy on Saturdays and Sundays. Even in large research hospitals, staffing is a problem with regard to both nurses and therapists. I am at ERH until June 15, 2023.

# 31

# Noise

Even though there's a lot less traffic between eleven at night and six in the morning, my end of the hallway is noisy with what seems like incessant hallway chatter. One patient, a white man, has had enough! I look out from my bed to glimpse and hear this man sitting up in his hospital bed, his belongings in tow, being whisked away down the hall, his bed rolling above the hallway speed limit. Like a rolling billboard, he announces his escape. "This place is like Grand Central Station. I've got to get outta here. I'm going to the other end of the hall." His parting message is directed at the nursing staff in the hallway, I'm sure. Everyone else is collateral damage. I detect no lies in his public announcement. Part of me wishes I'd thought of asking to be moved to another room, but if I had I wouldn't be present when my roommates need me.

I'm annoyed by the fact that my first hospital roommate, Ms. Brown, leaves the TV on at night. Its light rays disrupt the darkness; the sound compounds the hallway noise. On my first or second full day in the hospital, Dr. Milton stops by and asks, "How did you sleep?" Lying in a fetal position on my right side facing the curtain that separates my roommate's bed from my own, I point with my eyes and head in the direction of the TV mounted high up on wall, visible and audible from Ms. Brown's side of the room. Demonstrating compassion over my loss of sleep, Dr. Milton briefly places his hand around my left wrist and informs me in a low voice, so as not to offend Ms. Brown, "You know, all TVs are supposed to be turned off at 8:00 PM." This is news to me! Nobody told me, and there are no signs in the room about TV rules, at least none I ever see. Dr. Milton could have dismissed my complaint as one of the hazards of being in a hospital; but he doesn't. After he leaves the room, I am left to figure out how best to approach Ms. Brown.

I am a person who always means well, I think. I never intentionally try to harm another person, physically or with my words. Well, most of the time—my siblings, especially my older sister, Sina, and my brother Fred are exceptions. I remember popping Sina upside her head with a metal kitchen spatula shortly after we graduated from high school. We got into a scuffle after she wore, without my permission, a brand-new, expensive gray wool jumpsuit, which I'd purchased with my hard-earned money, and she stuffed it in the bottom of my closet like an old rag. Sina and I disagree about the reason for our fight. She says it was over a cookie; I seriously doubt it (smile). Anyway, I burst into tears and immediately regretted popping her after seeing that I broke skin. Siblings know how to press all the wrong (or right) buttons, the ones that turn Dr. Jekyll into Mr. Hyde.

I am new to the room; Ms. Brown was already here. She has not yet spoken a word to me. I decide to speak to her first. When she returns from morning therapy, I greet her,

"How are you, Ms. Brown? Did you have a good therapy session today?"

"I'm good. It was good, thank you," she replies.

I do not want my first words with Ms. Brown to be my request that she turn down the sound on her TV at night. I also don't want to hurt her feelings. Neither do I feel I should be forced to police and enforce the hospital rules.

Watching TV can be a means of self-medication, a way to take your mind off what ails or haunts you—trauma, sickness, loneliness, or something else. Thus, watching TV at night (or during the day) can become addictive, to the point that you cannot sleep or function without the TV on.

It's not that Ms. Brown's TV was abnormally or exceptionally loud the previous evening. The problem is that I am hypersensitive to unnecessary noise due to my stroke. The sound of the TV at night coupled with the hallway racket, my need to use the bed pan at least twice during the night, and the health care workers coming and going to draw blood or take vitals lessen my chances of getting a good night's sleep. I shift from side to side in the night and end up facing the light and sound from Ms. Brown's TV. It's less disruptive than the brightness and noise coming from the hallway. Too often the nurses come and go, leaving the door open at night. Sometimes I ask, "Would you please close the door on your way out?" Often before I can get the words out, the door is left open and the nurse is long gone. It's emotionally draining when you are sick.

"Ms. Brown, would you mind turning the sound on your TV lower at night. I'm unable to sleep."

"You don't like watching TV?" She turns the sound completely off; it is daytime.

"I didn't mean you should turn the TV off during the day. It just bothers me at night when I'm trying to sleep."

The TV remains on and the sound off, until Ms. Brown's boyfriend and sister visit her. Eventually, Ms. Brown turns the sound on her TV completely off, but only at night.

I read somewhere that we cannot recover or make up for lost sleep. My body is exhausted from lost sleep, the stroke, and energy expended in therapy. The first week when the therapists wheel me back to my room, they encourage me to stay in my wheelchair for fifteen minutes to an hour. "It's good for your lungs and back muscles," they advise. I believe them, but I cannot do it. I'm too uncomfortable sitting up in my wheelchair during that first week. I'm too weak; it's so painful. Shortly after the therapists leave after parking me in my room, I ask the nurse or nurse assistant to help me back into the bed. They never refuse.

One particular day when I'm dead asleep in my bed after expending all my energy in therapy, a nurse who sings and plays guitar stops in our room to entertain Ms. Brown and me. Our favorite nurse assistant Keisha had also stopped in to visit us. Later, Ms. Brown and Keisha tell me that I slept through the entire performance, which took place around three or so in the afternoon. "You didn't budge one inch," they report.

32

# A Shelterless Black Woman Cleans My Room

IF WE CANNOT IMAGINE a thing, somebody must imagine it for us and tell us about it until we can imagine or see it for ourselves. We depend on others to recognize or affirm our potential, especially when so much in the world says we have no potential, particularly as Black people and women. At ERH, the doctors and therapists first imagine what I cannot yet conceive for myself in this post-stroke body.

I'm not certain of the percentage, but from my limited perspective, it appears that all the patients on my floor are stroke victims. Our struggles are similar and different. We have various mobility and speech challenges, and we struggle with different cognitive and psychological difficulties. If the traffic that runs past my hospital room door is a correct indication, only one or two patients on my floor can walk the halls independently or with the assistance of a cane, walker, or hospital worker. We are not permitted out of our beds without calling for assistance; the bed rails are locked with alarms that go off if we attempt to leave our beds unassisted; these alarms are so loud that they cannot be ignored. Ask me how I know. I'll tell you about that later.

Illness and life itself are a complex intersectional equalizer. We enter the world as infants dependent upon other humans to do everything for us. Our parents teach us to be independent; our independence is considered a mark of maturity, the accomplishment of grown folk. Truth is, we are never not dependent on other people. And other humans depend on us; we are interdependent throughout our lives. We depend on others to dispose of the waste we create; to plant, harvest, transport, and market the foods we eat; to fight our wars; to clean the public bathrooms we use; to make our water drinkable; to care for us when we are ill, and so on and so on.

One day, I'm awake in my room when a Black woman enters with a broom and mop to clean the floors. Before she finishes, I thank her for cleaning my room. We talk as she sweeps and mops under my bed. I had lost one of the cylindrical-shaped red rubber grips with a hole through its center through which I force the handle of my spoon so I can hold it to feed myself. She spots it under the bed and uses the broom to retrieve it. I ask her name. Sadly, I don't remember it now. I'm one of those people who only remembers the names of people I meet for the first time if I see it in writing, especially if it's a unique name. The woman tells me that she is saving money to get her own place to live. Presently, the woman cleaning my room lives in a shelter for shelterless people. I am both surprised and disturbed by this revelation. I wish I had cash with me; I would tip her for cleaning my room. I tell her so. My room is clean because of her. I've visited many people in hospitals in my lifetime, including my mother. I've seen a lot of dirty hospital floors. My floor is spotless because of a shelterless Black woman.

## 33

# Occupational Therapy

I DEPEND ON THE occupational therapists to help and teach me how to do the mundane tasks I took for granted before my stroke but can no longer do for myself. Beth, an African American woman who has worked at Emory for about thirteen years, is one of my regular occupational therapists. Beth is an angel. She arrives early in the morning, around seven, and fills a yellow plastic basin with water to wash my body. The basin becomes my property; it is stored on my half of the cabinet to the left as you first enter my room. She wastes no time relinquishing to me part of the task of washing my body. The next morning, Beth retrieves my yellow plastic basin, fills it with warm water, places Bedside-Care Foam non-rinse cleanser in the water, draws the curtains around my bed, and lays out my towels, wash cloths, and clean scrubs. It's my turn to place the washcloth in the water and squeeze as much water out of it as I can manage and wash my body, beginning with my face. I have very little strength, but with each effort I improve, even if it doesn't seem so. The effect is accumulative. Since I cannot wash my back, Beth washes it and assists with putting on my deodorant, lotion, disposable underwear, and scrubs, and also with brushing my teeth. Nobody brushes my hair, except Lisa Weaver when she visits. My hair won't be washed until I'm home. After we finish washing and clothing my body, Beth helps me into my wheelchair and we travel to the large therapy room on the second floor.

## Reaching My Arms Up and Out

I seem to remember Dr. Milton asking me to extend my arms out in front of me as high as I could when I first met him. I couldn't extend my arms straight up over my head. I could only extend them a little higher than my shoulders. One of the first things Beth works on with me is reaching my arms out and upward. I'm surprised at how much energy it takes and how weak my arms and shoulders are. It's a very difficult range of motion for me. During the first week, Beth and I work on it quite a bit. She helps me out of my wheelchair and into a seated position on one of the exercise beds in the large therapy room. Next, she positions a large, tall board in front of me. It's like a rolling whiteboard except it has many uniform holes in it. My task is to place small pegs into the holes, as many as possible, reaching out high and low. It is a slow process at first. With this and other exercises that work similar muscles, the repetition awakens and strengthens my arm and back muscles, and my stamina improves.

## Water the Plants?!

Another one of my occupational therapists, an African American man called Michael (not his actual name), sometimes collects me in my wheelchair from my room and takes me to water all the plants in his work room. I absolutely do not look forward to watering his plants. I can't bear standing, even for short periods of time. I may have said to him, "Why don't you water your own plants?" I hate that he transports me to therapy on the second floor only to have me stand on my feet and water *his* plants! Michael insists that I pour water into both sides of each potted plant. I do it, but I fuss, under my breath, practically the entire time. *Just let the water flow around to the other side*, I think to myself. *All of them?! Water all the plants?! Save some for other patients to water. Better yet, do it yourself.* It feels like unnecessary torture.

Michael never wavers, despite my whining. I haven't yet made the connection between our seemingly gratuitous plant-watering sessions and the plants that will need my care when I'm back home alone. My condition doesn't let me think that far ahead. But my therapists do. Independent living is not a thing I can yet imagine. As my back and leg muscles grow stronger and my balance improves, I appreciate and understand why Michael has insisted that I water his umpteen plants. I also eventually realize how the many exercises that I practice with Beth and the plant-watering sessions with Michael reinforce each other; both are meant to strengthen or awaken the muscles in my arms, back, and legs.

## Cards and Games

Beth and Michael assemble me and two other patients in a room for a group therapy session where we play a card game. I'd never heard of the game, much less played it before, and don't remember its name. None of us patients know how to play the game. Michael plays it very well. Of course he does, since he plays the game often with patients. Michael joins the game with us, which bothers me. Michael wins every game! My attitude is *That's not fair*. Persnickety me asks Beth, who doesn't play but simply coaches from the sideline, "Why is he playing with us?" She responds, "You're funny." However, I'm not trying to be funny; I'm always rooting for the underdog. And I'm one of the underdogs in this game! *It's fine and necessary that the therapists instruct us, but let us play among ourselves*, I reason to myself. I want one of us to win the game. All the patients lose while the therapist wins. *That's not good for patient morale*, I complain to myself. Beth says, "I would never take you to a card game with me." I don't have a poker face. Quite the opposite; everybody knows what I'm holding or not holding.

It's the same situation with another game I've played in a group therapy session, except two white women therapists, Sue and Kathy (not their actual names), are playing against two or three patients, including me. The therapists help us with the rules and provide tips. Either Sue or Kathy always wins the game. In fact, Sue announces before we begin, "Kathy always wins this game." What fun is that? When I finally figure out the game and begin doing well, I provide pointers or clues to the young Latino patient so he might win a game. He seems more cognitively and physically challenged than me. He thanks me for my help. When he wins, I feel like a winner too.

# 34

# Speech Therapy

From my conversations with the speech therapists and based on the early tests that they give me, I did not incur any damage to my speech or cognition as a result of my stroke. The speech therapists want to ensure that I am at my pre-stroke level of cognition. I play a lot of cognitive games in speech therapy; most of the earlier games seem tedious and unhelpful. But I play. A skill that I work on at ERH (and in outpatient therapy after I'm discharged) is the ability to avoid being distracted while performing certain tasks and to recall information received after being distracted. I find that I am easily distracted at times. We work on concentration and memory to make sure that I'm where I was before the stroke. The game that I remember playing most often involves selecting a card from a stack. On each card, a list of clues is provided for arranging twelve colored chips in boxes printed on the square cardboard. Each card is also labeled to reflect the level of difficulty. The higher the number, the more difficult the exercise. I am to place the chips in a certain order on the playing board within the boxes printed on it. There are three vertical boxes and four horizontal ones, giving a total of twelve boxes within the square. A card might, for example, instruct the player to "Select 3 red chips, 3 blue, 2 black, 3 orange, and 1 white." Based on clues on the card, the player must then position the colored chips so that each one ends up in a specific position on the card in relation to the other chips. For example, it might read "Place the white chip to the left of an orange chip but not above a red chip" and so on until all twelve chips are in their correct spaces. If one is not placed in the correct space or box, others cannot be placed in the proper box. When I finish, the therapist examines what I've done and asks me to explain. If I make a mistake, 99 percent of the time I self-correct while listening to my explanation of why I ordered the chips as I did. Within thirty to forty minutes, I usually complete four or five games. As I advance in levels of difficulty, I enjoy the challenge of the game. I think we started at a medium level of difficulty.

One day, my regular therapist, Sandy (not her actual name), is unavailable. I meet with another speech therapist. In the room with us is a white male doctor. He is sitting at the table with us, opposite me. I am facing him, but he is facing his computer. Feels rude to me. The speech therapist, a white woman, is sitting next to and facing my left shoulder. I cannot recall the exercise she has us doing but I remember completing it correctly and in record time, according to her. Suddenly, the man, who has not introduced himself, stops typing on his computer and turns to me. "Something told me I should pay attention to you. You are doing quite well with the exercise, better than other patients. You are special." I hope all the patients are seen as special. Turns out he is a medical doctor, and he supervises the speech therapists, as I remember. He has been on sick leave, which is why I've never met him before. This is his first day back on the job. He asks me about my education and what I do for a living. He too is a Christian, a fairly new one. As he talks about being a believer, he strikes me as a fundamentalist Christian. I'm telling myself not to be judgmental. I listen and try to respond very little. I don't want to offend or encourage him to keep talking. He mentions the name of a man who discipled him; I'm not familiar with him. He asks me a theological question (that I cannot recall) and wants to know my thoughts. I'm very hesitant. I'm here for therapy, and the young woman, the speech therapist, hasn't signed up for this conversation. She is quiet. I'm uncomfortable. I remember responding, "You probably don't want to hear what I think on that topic. I'm quite progressive. Some might call me radical." But he sincerely wants to know what I think. I look at the woman again. I don't want to monopolize her time talking about religion, but I accommodate him. He listens and is quite humble. The next day he comes to my room early before Dr. Justin and Dr. Milton arrive to make their daily rounds.

"I want to thank you for our conversation yesterday. It gave me peace. You really blessed me." As I write this in my memoir, I wish I remembered the topic of our conversation, but I do not. "I got word that my father had died. Our conversation helped me cope with that news." We did not talk about death, I'm certain.

"I'm so glad our conversation was helpful to you. I'm so sorry about your father. Thank you for telling me," I offer. I am truly thankful that he feels that I've been helpful to him. Dealing with a serious illness, I sometimes feel like life is passing me by. Every time I see him in the hallway, he greets me, "Hi, Dr. Smith."

## 35

# Physical Therapy and Walking

WHEN I LEFT EH, I had learned to stand up and walk maybe fifteen to twenty steps with the help of a walker and accompanied by the therapist. At ERH, I receive a wheelchair. Surprisingly, my legs are stronger than I imagined. I'm able to push the wheelchair along with my legs, but not with my hands. My arms and hands are too weak to grab and push the wheels. During the first five days of physical therapy, I practice standing up and sitting down from the wheelchair. Eventually, I am able to stand up, put my hands on the walker, and walk a few steps from my wheelchair to the threshold of the large therapy room, which is about ten steps there and back. We also practice walking up the three steps on the staircase. Over ten to twelve therapy sessions, I progress from one trip up the three steps and back down to being able to go up and down the staircase two or three times. In the same period of time, I advance from walking a few steps in the therapy room, to walking the long hallway on the therapy floor, to walking in the back courtyard and up a slight incline with the walker. A couple days before I'm discharged, I'm walking the steps necessary to stop receiving the painful anticoagulant shots in my lower stomach. Two days before my discharge, I'm strong enough to abandon the wheelchair and the walker for a wide thick belt around my waist that the therapist can hold so that she can prevent me from falling should I lose my balance. I find that I'm very good at losing my balance without falling. I teeter to the right at about a thirty-degree angle with my left leg up in the air about half a foot off the floor, but I eventually regain balance, placing my left foot back on the ground. I'm elated when the therapist finally puts me on the stationary bike. Riding the stationary bike, the muscles in my legs, thighs, and calves come to life, and I feel my lungs becoming stronger. I graduate from pushing my wheelchair along with my legs, to standing behind it and pushing it, to walking the hallway with the walker, and finally, to walking with the belt around my waist accompanied by the therapist or a nurse. When Michael asks me if I'd like to go outside, I am excited because I haven't been outside since I was admitted to the ICU at Emory. I miss the sunshine and fresh air. He wheels me outside and we sit on a bench near a table in the sun. "Do you think you can walk around the table once?" he asks. "I'll try," I reply. A walk about the table with the walker is about six or eight steps. I make the trip once and sit down. Eventually, I'm able to go around the table twice. Stacey, the physical therapist, also takes me outside, and I walk to the little mosquito-infested garden where we rest awhile before walking back to my wheelchair. Soon, I am walking from the door that leads back into the hospital from the courtyard to the elevators while Stacey pushes my wheelchair. It is a slow, difficult trek but I make it. I'm exhausted afterwards and anxious to sit back down in my wheelchair. Some regulars at the reception desk witness my progress and often let me know how well I'm doing. Stacey pushes me a little further with each session. I've had fourteen sessions in fourteen days.

## Walking

One day, while lying in my bed, something strange, something I've never experienced before, happens. I see myself, a duplicate me, rolling or scooting my body across the bed, placing my feet on the floor, and starting to walk in the direction of Ms. Brown's bed. I don't know if what I'm watching is a daydream, *déjà vu*, a vision, my spirit, or my ghost. In those brief seconds, I'm still aware of my physical body. The sight lasts less than ten seconds. The possibility that I might try to follow this apparition frightens me—I know I would fall—I cannot walk. Writing this memoir is the first time I've thought about that experience since the day it happened.

My mother never stopped believing that God would heal her legs; she would walk again during her lifetime. Her faith was the *sine qua non* (the indispensable ingredient) of her hope. Doctors and hospitals gave her none. She never walked again. She could live without walking but not without the hope that she would walk.

## Physical Therapy and Walking

I love sitting on the side of my hospital bed forcing my feet into my size six Merrell tennis shoes, which are designed with a bright yellow, orange, lime green, lavender, and purple rainbow pattern on a gray-and-blue-speckled canvas. People say, "I love your tennis shoes." I love putting on my tennis shoes during the day. During the night, my feet go from numb to excruciatingly painful. I call the nurse for painkillers so that I can sleep. ERH doesn't want patients in unnecessary pain; I'm so thankful.

Initially, the nurse asks, "Would you like some Tylenol?"

"No, Tylenol didn't help at home. I need something stronger."

The nurse contacts the doctor for permission to give me a painkiller. Subsequently, she administers a half dose (0.5 tablets of a 2.5 mg) of oxycodone every six hours during the night. Despite the numbness in my feet during the day, wearing my tennis shoes and pushing my wheelchair with my feet stimulates my feet. My feet need movement and want to walk, which gives me hope that I will walk again.

# 36

# Meal Plan

I DISCOVER THAT MY hospital chart instructs the nurses or nurse assistants to weigh me daily. I am weighed two to three times during my sixteen days at ERH. I still can't handle much food, and the poor quality of the food doesn't help. The quiche fools me once but not twice. It is bright yellow, has a perfectly tanned crust, and spinach visible throughout. When I bite into it, it has the texture of papier mâché and the taste of cardboard. How does one go so wrong with quiche?! Generally, I don't eat red meat or pork, but I must eat to survive and at least maintain my famished body frame. So I order the steak one day for dinner. To say it tastes and feels like leather is an understatement. And I never ever imagined that anyone could ruin a boiled egg. Live long enough and anything is possible. Bananas, scrambled eggs, pork bacon, bites of mashed potatoes (can't take too much), spaghetti (the least dry dinner option), a scrawny salad, lemon or raspberry ice, and chocolate Ensure become my food staples. The nurses constantly remind me that I must have a bowel movement, or they'll give me an enema. I assure them I will when I am able to consume enough eatable food. I do my best. God knows, I don't want an enema. An enema might confuse my body organs for waste, I fear.

Other than the lemon and raspberry ice and the Ensure, I don't crave, desire, or tolerate processed sweets. The applesauce at ERH tastes too sweet, unlike the applesauce at EH. I ask the woman who delivers my meals, "Do you all have any no-sugar-added applesauce?" "The applesauce you get here *is* no-sugar-added," she says. I am flummoxed. All I know is that I am repulsed by the applesauce; it tastes entirely too sweet. I have become hypersensitive to unnatural sweets or refined sugar. I believe this hypersensitivity has saved my teeth from tooth decay. If the nurse assistants or nurses do not remember to brush my teeth or don't have the time, they go unbrushed until I learn to brush them myself. Still, I need the staff to at least hand me my toothbrush. My teeth are never flossed during my hospitalization because I don't have the dexterity or strength in my fingers.

# 37

# Lucky

I AM LUCKY, YES lucky, that the stroke doesn't seem to have impacted my cognitive abilities. It seems my speech is not diminished either. I also have no paralysis except in my toes, perhaps. Many Christians shame other Christians for describing themselves as lucky. Every good thing must be expressed in the language of blessing, and blessings only come from God. I don't feel obligated to use that language. I don't believe God is so easily offended by language, despite how writers of biblical texts sometimes characterize God as vindictive, narcissistic, and jealous. In both the Hebrew Bible/Old Testament and the Second/New Testament, writers testify that God doesn't show favoritism toward one people over another.[1] Of course, there are individuals in the Bible who are characterized as making the same claim, such as Mary, the mother of Jesus of Nazareth (Luke 1:48). But Christians often insist that their "blessings" are the result of God's special favor precisely because they are Christians. And they are often offended when other Christians don't use the same language to describe their experiences. It's not that I don't use the words "bless" and "blessings" as a verb and a noun, respectively, to reflect God's actions. I just don't believe God is in any way limited by or confined to the language of the Bible or human language. I don't believe that certain words or any one language, including the ancient languages in which the Bible was written, are inherently sacred

---

1. For example, Deut 10:17; Gal 2:6. Women of the civil rights movement like Fannie Lou Hamer relied on Acts 17:26 to support their belief in racial and women's equality. It speaks to the common ancestry of all human beings.

or most sacred. In fact, the division between the sacred and the secular is a human construct, just as human languages are created by humans for humans, not for God. I don't believe that God favors me more than people who have strokes that result in one side of their bodies being paralyzed or in slurred speech or diminished cognitive ability. I don't believe that God favors the person who never suffers a stroke above me. I don't believe that the person who dies of a stroke died because God took them. I believe life happens to all of us, and that systems and structures, as well as personal and familial decisions and habits, impact our quality of life. We can only control those things within our control. I cannot revise my family history of stroke and its inevitable impact on my life. I can only make better choices that might mitigate the impact of the risk that my family history poses.

God has given us free will, which gives me a lot of control over my own life. My decisions and actions impact other people and society. God is not a puppeteer who pulls the strings that control my every movement or thought on the stage of life on which we perform and where we do battle with personal, spiritual, and systemic forces. I think allegiance to the word "blessing" comes primarily from a worship of the language of the Bible as translated into English and from a prosperity gospel that has infiltrated religion and churches. God is neither limited to nor controlled by our human language choices, even those in the various Bible translations. That's a whole other problem. Toni Morrison asks a question worth pondering: "Is it possible to write religion-inflected prose narrative that does not rest its case entirely or mainly on biblical language? Is it possible to make the experience and journey of faith fresh, as new and as linguistically unencumbered as it was to early believers, who themselves had no collection of books to rely on?"[2]

I am lucky to be at ERH where Dr. Milton is the attending physician. It is a known fact that African American patients do not always receive compassionate care from white doctors and nurses.[3] Dr. Milton is not the typical white doctor that many Black people and other people of color encounter. He is very cordial and friendly, and he compassionately touches his patients on the arm or hand, as he did me. Of all the doctors in the

---

2. Morrison, *Source of Self-Regard*, 253.

3. According to Stephanie Cornish, "The researchers found that when doctors were interacting with White patients, for example, they would stand at the patient's bedside and were more likely to touch the invalid in a sympathetic way. When the doctors interacted with the Black patients, however, they would stand by the door holding their binder." See Cornish, "Black Patients Treated with Less Compassion Than Whites."

Emory system who visit me in my room at EH or ERH, Dr. Milton and Dr. Justin stand in closest proximity to me when at my hospital bed. I get the impression that Dr. Milton doesn't meet a stranger in his hospital. Like me, Dr. Milton came to Georgia from the Detroit area. He doesn't spend much time with his patients (the nature of the health care beast), but he seems genuinely interested in his patients when he is with them. Beth, my occupational therapist, speaks well of Dr. Milton, and when she does her fondness and respect for him radiates in the tone of her voice and the smile on her face. I only hear good things about him from the hospital staff.

Sometime after leaving the hospital, I search for Dr. Milton on the internet. I'm curious to know where he received his medical training. I'm surprised to learn that he earned his medical degree from Howard University School of Medicine, the Harvard of HBCUs, and he did his residency at Howard University Hospital. Makes sense! Ironically, HBCUs don't possess the billions or hundreds of millions of dollars of the Ivy League schools, whose endowments come from their involvement in the enslavement of Black people.

Dr. Milton also has great internet reviews, with most reviewers testifying that his bedside manner is excellent and that Emory is "lucky to have him." I concur. The only complaints are about the limited time the reviewers have with him; he's in demand. I'm unable to schedule a four-week follow-up with him after I'm discharged because he has no appointments until six months out.

It matters where and how doctors are trained to interact with patients. In my experience, Dr. Justin is not the type of doctor to touch a patient as a show of compassion, but he demonstrates human care and compassion in other ways. At some point, the doctors tell me that my potassium is low and start me on a potassium intravenous drip. It burns so badly that all I can do is curl up on my left side and stare into the darkness of the room as tears stream down my cheeks and hushed cries escape my lips. Dr. Justin enters my room. His voice announces his presence.

"Dr. Smith, we need to extend the potassium drip for another day. Do you think you can hang in there?"

"If I have to, I will," I respond after turning my head to the right to look at him, my face wet with tears.

"I'll contact the doctor [I assume Dr. Milton] to see if we can give you the potassium pills instead and stop the drip."

"Okay."

The next day the nurse removes the drip, and another large pill is added to the many meds I'm already taking. I never imagined I'd be taking prescription meds for a serious chronic illness.

# 38

# Doctor in the House?

NONE OF MY NURSES or my hospital roommates know that I'm a professor with an earned PhD. Illness is or can be an equalizer. Illness and health care are inflected or complicated by race, gender, ethnicity, ableness, poverty, sexuality, geography, and sometimes religion. The nurses and nurse assistants don't know me as Dr. Smith until Dr. Clarice Martin (the first black woman to earn a PhD in New Testament) calls the hospital reception desk on the third floor looking for me.

"I'm looking for Dr. Smith, a patient in your hospital."

*"We don't have a doctor as a patient here."*

"Yes, you do. Her name is Dr. Mitzi Smith," Clarice insists.

*"Oh, we didn't know she is a doctor."*

All of a sudden, I am a celebrity, at least in the eyes of one Black woman, a charge nurse, and this makes me uncomfortable. I don't want to be treated better or worse than anyone else. But I'm also pleased that I can make a Black woman proud. She cares for me with respect and compassion before and after that little revelation. No one knows, however, that I earned my PhD at Harvard University until a young white male doctoral student from Boston University asks me where I earned my doctorate in an exit interview the day before I'm discharged.

Before Clarice's call, I don't realize that I have a phone in my hospital room. I didn't see it; nobody told me it was there; it is not plugged in. Clarice's call moves me deeply. I'm flattered when she says, "They don't know who they have in their hospital! But they know now." I'm mostly grateful that she took the time to call me and that she expresses sincere concern for my well-being. Clarice fears that I will be gone too soon, like Dr. Cain Hope Felder, who died on October 1, 2019, at the age of seventy-six at his home in Mobile, Alabama. Felder was Clarice's contemporary, my mentor at Howard Divinity School, and a pioneering African American biblical scholar. He edited and contributed to the first academic book on African American biblical interpretation, *Stony the Road We Trod*.

My mother was the first to imagine I could earn a PhD. She'd say, "You should go get a PhD." "A PhD in what?" My mother attended a Black high school in Cleveland, Tennessee. Despite her scars and narcolepsy, she was valedictorian of her graduating class. In high school, she studied two years of Latin and two years of French. I studied no languages at Central High School in Columbus, Ohio, which was a segregated but predominantly white school.

Felder was the first person who said to me, "You should consider a PhD in New Testament." After completing my three-year master of divinity degree at Howard University School of Divinity, I remained an extra year to study Latin, Middle Egyptian Hieroglyphs, and French and German reading in the university's classics department in preparation for applying to doctoral programs.

Clarice promises, "Our entire church will be praying for you this Sunday." I am always happy for the prayers of sincere, humble people. On my worst days and my best days, I believe somebody's praying for me. I try to be that somebody for someone else.

Part 3: Fighting My Way Back

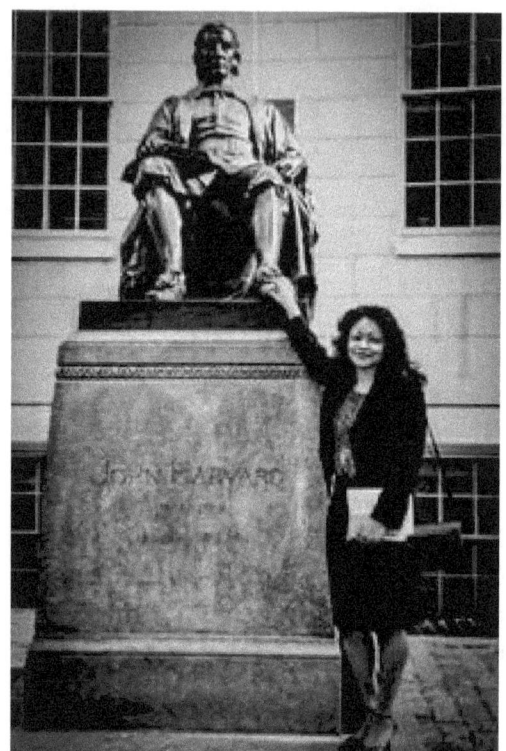

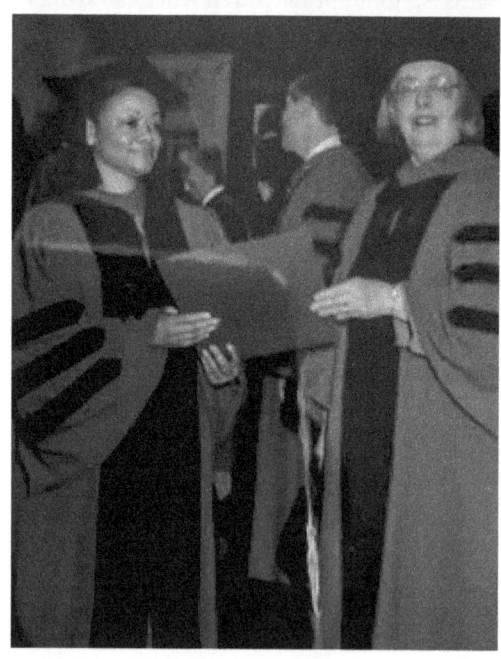

# 39

# Paul and Georgia

THE APOCALYPTIC BOOK OF Revelation demonstrates that angels can be rebellious, combative, and death-dealing, and they can even engage in war (in heaven no less! See Rev 12:7). Like humans, they err. On a scale of created beings, they are like humans (e.g., they speak human language, wear human clothing, and look like men); they seem more than human; and they are less than God. As mentioned earlier, it's interesting—but not shocking, given the patriarchal nature of the Bible—that all the angels named in the Bible and in apocryphal texts are gendered male, the most famous being Gabriel. Yet ironically, in our modern society, we seldom refer to grown men as angelic. That adjective is reserved for children, regardless of their gender, and women. Not all angels are helpful, liberating, and therapeutic or facilitators of peace and wholeness. But they are angels, nonetheless.

Similar to EH, not all the nurses who care for me at ERH are consistently good, and some are rarely or never good or compassionate toward me. They are all angels to me, but some have lost their way, maybe due to their own battles with physical illness, age, social and institutional oppressions, and so forth. Human beings and angels are complex. We may start with the best of intentions, but something goes awry that we just can't shake off as we stumble through life and when we enter our places of employment and other spaces.

## Paul and Mrs. Masai

One health care worker may be a troublesome and even harmful angel to me but a good and helpful angel to another person. After Ms. Brown is discharged, Mrs. Masai (not her actual name) becomes my new roommate. She was a hospice worker before her stroke, which occurred during brain surgery. Mrs. Masai responds very little to the doctors, nurses, or therapists. When she speaks to me, it is usually to say one or two words: "Reposition" or "Help me." When she says "reposition," I know to push the button and call for help: "Mrs. Masai, the patient in bed B, needs to be repositioned in her bed." Mrs. Masai becomes more animated and talkative when her two sons, her daughter-in-law, and her husband visit. They arrive bearing containers of homemade Kenyan food. She communicates robustly with her family in Kiswahili. Paul, my problematic male nurse, is sometimes Mrs. Masai's night nurse. But he also visits Mrs. Masai on nights when he is not her nurse. When he visits her, he turns on the light on my side of the room, leaves his nurse's cart at the foot of my bed, and enters behind the curtain that separates Mrs. Masai from me. His visits are usually around 11:30 at night or later. Paul never turns on the light on Mrs. Masai's side of the curtain/room. Fed up with being disturbed late at night, I finally confront him.

"Paul, would you please take your cart with you into Mrs. Masai's side of the room and turn her light on instead of mine so that I might better attempt to sleep."

"It's just easier for me," he responds.

As unhelpful and disrespectful as Paul is to me, he is very helpful to Mrs. Masai. He explains things to her in their native language in great detail, if the length of the conversation is any indication. And she is quite talkative with him, even more so than when her family visits. She comes to life. Perhaps the questions she would ask the doctors, she reserves for Paul because it's easier to ask in her native tongue after a stroke. A stroke can cause regression to an earlier stage of life. Mrs. Masai doesn't speak with the physical therapists who come to help her out of bed and into her wheelchair except to say, "Don't want to," "No," or "Reposition." So I guess Paul, the thorn in my side, is her good angel.

## Georgia

God is no respecter of persons, unlike people, institutions, and systems. At Emory Rehab, my room has no shower, just a sink and toilet, which is also shared with an adjoining room. We learn to wash ourselves from a small yellow plastic basin. My roommates cannot wash themselves due to paralysis, so they receive bed baths. Evidently, some hospital rooms in the newer section of ERH have showers. I haven't had a shower for about two weeks when a part-time nurse named Georgia arrives in my room around six one morning. I know Georgia. She has served as my nurse on other occasions. Georgia is not my nurse on the day she offers me a shower.

"Would you like a shower this morning?"

"How you gonna to do that?"

"Don't worry about it, let me take care of that. Do you want one?"

"Yes."

"Okay. Let me get everything ready, and I will be back."

"Okay."

This is my lucky day! It's Georgia's habit, and hers alone, to treat three patients with varying degrees of mobility challenges to a hot shower whenever she comes to work at ERH. She works at some other prestigious health care facility during the day, I'm told.

About half an hour later, Georgia returns to help me into my wheelchair. First, we stop in the small storage room where we find stacks of clean, light blue hospital scrubs neatly arranged on shelves. Georgia searches and finally finds a coveted size small bottoms but only a medium top. (Heretofore, I've been wearing medium bottoms and tops, which are way too big for me.) Next, Georgia rolls me down the hall and around the corner past the elevators on the left and the reception desk on the right, before we take a hard left down the hall turning away from the reception desk. About halfway down the long hallway to the left, we enter what looks to be an old, small group shower room. Georgia has already efficiently laid out the white towels, wash cloths, and soap, and she's positioned the shower chair in the shower. Closing the door behind us, Georgia turns the shower on, tests the water temperature with her hand, and helps me out of my wheelchair and onto the shower stool. The warm water cascading over my skin feels heavenly; I don't want to leave. But Georgia has two other patients to shower; I must go. When the shower is complete, Georgia dresses me quickly and rolls me back to my room. On our return, the nurse at the reception desk says, "You look so refreshed and happy, Ms. Smith." "I am. Thank you. I am," I respond with my biggest smile since my stroke. That is a shower I will never forget and for which I'm eternally grateful to Georgia!

The next day, Georgia returns to give Ms. Brown a shower.

Georgia is one of my angels. God is like Georgia. Georgia is like God. God works miracles for and among humans in collaboration with human beings, I believe. Human beings collaborate with God to create miracles. I wish we'd do it all the time and in every space, or at least more often.

# 40

# Tears

EVERY ACT OF COMPASSION helps the healing process and mitigates the abuse and mistreatment that I and other patients experience from some hurtful, cruel, hurting, and overworked health care workers. An instance of abuse that I experience during my first or second week at ERH is perpetrated by Janice (not her actual name), a nurse assistant, a Black woman, perhaps a little younger than me. I can't identify her specific country of origin but her accent sounds Caribbean, although from which island I cannot tell. My longtime friend and college roommate, Donna, who is a wonderful nurse herself, is from Jamaica. Donna and my now deceased Trinidadian good friend Kenneth Mulzac (we all went to the same Adventist college in Takoma Park, Maryland) would chide me, "Jamaicans and Trinidadians don't sound the same."

At about one in the morning, I push the call button because I need the bed pan to pee. Janet arrives and puts me on the pan.

"Why are you taking so long?!"

I finish and Janet removes the pan. "You pee too much. What's wrong with you?" She summons Nurse Paul, yes, problematic Paul. "She is peeing too much. Something is wrong with her."

"Nothing is wrong with me.... They gave me a diuretic." I'm certain it must be in the chart. If they'd look at the chart.

Following Janet's lead, Paul responds, "What's wrong with you? You in pain?"

"No! I have sense enough to say if I'm in pain!" I'm pissed. "It's 1:00 AM. Just empty the bed pan?! And leave me alone," I insist.

Janet finally empties the bed pan and leaves. She returns later to deliver a snide remark in her native dialect. I can't translate her words but recognize the condescending tone. "What's the matter?! You can't understand my language?!" That night I curl up and cry. I realize that I'm at the mercy of a woman capable of being mean and cruel to her patients. I depend on her for my care throughout the night. I cannot go to the toilet on my own. I hold my urine for as long as I can before calling for assistance. And when I call, I have to call several times before she comes to help me onto the bed pan again, even though, based on the chatter in the hallway, she's not far away. I hope I don't have to pee again until the morning shift change.

My roommate Ms. Brown was also brought to tears by the dehumanizing words and actions of health care workers. I must have finally fallen into a deep sleep that night. Sleepless hospital nights can accumulate until one day or night you fall into a deep sleep that no one and nothing can disturb, except the phlebotomist maybe. The body can only take so many sleepless nights before it takes matters into its own hands, for better or for worse. Evidently, a nurse or nurse assistant had taken Ms. Brown's clothes off to change her for bed but was called away to an emergency situation elsewhere on the floor. No one returned to put Ms. Brown into her pajamas or pull the covers over her. She was left all night unclothed in the frigid air conditioning. (We are constantly asking somebody to turn the air conditioning down.)

Early the next morning, Ms. Brown reports to the therapist who shows up to help her, the charge nurse, or both how she was left practically naked all night. She cannot tell it without sobbing. "Do you want to file a claim about the incident ?" "No." Ms. Brown fears retaliation. Retaliation is real, as I discovered when I was at EH. When Ms. Brown's 7:00 AM shift nurse assistant, a young African American woman, arrives (my day nurse is also present writing something on my wall chart in front of me), Ms. Brown breaks down sobbing again as she recounts to her how she was left in the cold overnight without any clothes on. "She talked to me like I'm not even a human being," Ms. Brown adds. This is the first I'm hearing this part of the story. Now I'm also in tears. Unfortunately, both the nurse and the nurse assistant in the room demonstrate little to no empathy for Ms. Brown, neither by their words nor their actions. Instead, like politicians, they rehearse talking points: the nurses have so many patients; sometimes they get called away on emergencies; they may intend to return but something else happens. As I sit on my bed watching and listening, I am deeply disturbed by the excuses and callousness. Neither of them moves closer to Ms. Brown or touches her while she cries uncontrollably.

"Ms. Brown, if I could get up out of this bed, I would come over there and hug you," I interject into the silence that follows the litany of excuses. The young African American nurse assistant who is standing near Ms. Brown the whole time finally puts her arm on her shoulder in a show of compassion. The fact that the nurses are understaffed or are called away is not Ms. Brown's problem. She still needs and deserves humane health care and empathy when the system and the people in it fail her.

This incident happens the day before Ms. Brown is discharged from the hospital. When her family arrives to take her home, she doesn't tell them what happened because she doesn't want to upset them. Ironically, the next time a nurse assistant shows such an egregious lack of empathy toward me is also the day before I go home.

# 41

# Visitors

IN THE ICU I couldn't have visitors. At EH I did not want a lot of visitors yet. I was still trying to wrap my mind around what was happening in my body. I had no tolerance for a lot questions. I know that people mean well but answering the same questions over and over is draining. I needed all the energy I could muster to focus on surviving. As I've stated, people would text me asking "How are you?" *How do you think I am after a stroke?!* I'd think. *I'm still fighting for my life.*

My state of mind—my intolerance for other people's need to know and their need for updates about my condition while I'm fighting for my life—reminds me of a conversation I had with my mother sometime before she died. I told her that I wanted to be with her when she took her last breath.

"Don't you want me to be there, Mommy?"

"No."

"No? What?! Why not?!"

"Because I'll be talking to God. My mind will be elsewhere."

I wanted to be at Mommy's bedside; she didn't need me there. I didn't want her to be alone. She believed she wouldn't be alone; God would be there. I was not there when my mother took her last breath. It still hurts. It also hurt when I left home and my mother's side for the first time in my life. Mommy and Anna Slocum, best friends and both physically challenged (a stroke paralyzed one side of Anna's body; my mother was confined to a wheelchair without a definitive diagnosis), made sure I boarded a Greyhound bus from Columbus, Ohio, to Takoma Park, Maryland, to attend Columbia Union College (CUC) to earn a BA in theology. My baby sister Lenora (eight years younger) and I wept. I called my mother as soon as possible the next day after my midnight arrival. I wept again when I called home from the dormitory phone booth and Mommy said, "I just want you to be happy." The very next day, I landed a job at the headquarters of the Seventh-day Adventist Church (less than two miles from CUC) as a part-time secretary receiving a student's wage, despite my two-year associate's degree in applied business (legal secretarial science) and three years of experience as a legal secretary/paralegal. God's Spirit plus my ability to send money home gave me peace.

I have no close family members in Georgia or nearby. They all live in Columbus. When family members live from paycheck to paycheck, they can't afford to take time off from work, even when emergencies arise. Illness costs everyone. My sister Sina and my eighteen-year-old grandniece, Napria, arrive to see me when they are able, no sooner and no later.

I'm suspicious that Napria is most interested in sightseeing around Atlanta and visiting friends, but she assures me that she has arrived to help. I soon discover that a friend of hers is going off to college in Florida, and she plans to visit him before he leaves and they won't see each other again for a long time. Napria is anxious to drive my 2021 black Honda Civic Sport, which she convinced me to purchase after I had gifted her my 2014 Honda Accord. She is a responsible driver, but I refused to let her drive into downtown Atlanta after 10:00 PM. In her youthful wishful thinking, she thinks she will eventually own the Civic too. Nevertheless, Napria is very helpful during her stay. She clips my toenails, which hadn't been trimmed since I entered the ER weeks ago. Next morning, she offers to make French toast for breakfast. But I don't eat or buy white bread.

"Don't you have any white bread?" she asks in disbelief.

"No, but there's some whole grain bread in the fridge."

"Whoever heard of making French toast with wheat bread?! You can't make French toast with wheat bread," she insists.

"Of course you can," I respond. I'm agitated now.

We go back and forth, as I get more and more frustrated. Finally, I turn away from her in the kitchen, and lie down on my makeshift bed in the living room, deciding to mind my own business. "Do whatever you want, girl."

Napria finally resigns herself to use the wheat bread, making the French toast and serving it to me.

"This is so good, Pria! What did you put in the French toast?" I ask.

Napria beams with pride, and immediately texts her friends and calls her mother to tell them that Aunt Mitty said I made the best French toast she ever tasted. Turns out she added some vanilla extract and cinnamon to her egg batter.

Between and after Sina and Napria's visits, I'm grateful for my friends and colleagues at Columbia Theological Seminary (CTS) who visit: Drs. Lisa Weaver, Christine Yoder, Raj Nadella, and Ralph Watkins, as well as the trustee board chair, attorney Jane Fahey. Lisa and Christine alternate their visits while I'm at ERH.

When CTS student Samantha Kendrick visits, she graciously plucks the wild hairs from my chin. It's interesting the things we do and don't concern ourselves with when we are seriously ill and as we recover. Lisa Weaver had braided the hair on top of my head in cornrows, since I cannot comb my hair. Samantha unbraids the cornrows, because I feel they are messy now. The nurses tell me that they liked my hair as it was. I roll my eyes, but only in my mind.

# 42

# Two Days Before I'm Discharged
## I Still Need Help!

IN MY LAST TWO days at ERH, I have three memorable bathroom experiences: one is very hurtful, and the other two are hilarious (at least I think so). Two days before ERH discharges me, I'm approved to walk to the bathroom with the therapy belt around my waist. But I must always call for assistance so that a nurse is with me to prevent me from falling in case I lose my balance. My balance is not good.

### Hurtful Bathroom Experience

I'm right-handed but my right hand is weak, numb, and lacks agility. I cannot feel the toilet paper in my right hand, let alone my butt. I can't feel anything with my right hand. After using the toilet, I must try cleaning myself with my left hand. So I always need assistance. The day before I'm discharged from ERH is no exception. Just before 7:00 AM, before a shift change, I need to use the toilet. I call for help, and my nurse assistant buckles the therapy belt around my waist and watches me go into the bathroom. After I finish using the toilet, I start wiping my butt with my left hand. I look to see if the toilet paper is clean. It is not, no matter how much I wipe. *I must have diarrhea*, I think. I don't want to leave the bathroom with a dirty bottom—nobody does. I hit the help button on the wall to my left.

"I need help."

"Okay, I'll send your nurse." A new shift has begun. My nurse assistant for the day, a Black woman about my age, comes into the bathroom door through the adjoining room. No one is in that room because the air conditioning isn't working properly.

"What do you need?" the nurse assistant asks, standing in the doorway.

"I need help cleaning myself."

Before I can explain that I have diarrhea and am not sure that I'm clean yet, she yells, "You are going home tomorrow. You should be able to wipe yourself by now!"

I'm hurt, angry, and loud now. "If you don't want to help me, leave."

"I didn't say I don't want to help you," she argues.

I've already pushed the help button again. Our conversation can probably be heard over the intercom now. "You might as well have. Leave me alone! I'll get somebody else."

My nurse, a young African American woman, enters the bathroom and sends the nurse assistant out. "How can I help you, Ms. Smith?"

"I need help cleaning myself."

In less than ten minutes, the nurse patiently and thoroughly cleans my bottom. Maya Angelou famously said, "People will forget what you said, people will forget what you did, but people will never forget how you made them feel." I will never forget how that nurse assistant made me feel, how she shamed me. Many stroke survivors are discharged from hospitals in worse condition than me, able to do very little for themselves. Yes, I'm going home, but I still have a long road to full recovery, if there is such a thing as a *full* recovery.

## Hilarious Bathroom Experiences

The first amusing experience happens after I've graduated from sitting in the wheelchair, to walking with the walker, and finally to walking with the therapy belt around my waist. Lying in my bed, I call for the nurse or nurse assistant to accompany me to the bathroom. Nobody comes for too long a period of time, and I've got to go. So I scoot my body down toward the end of the bed where there's a space between the protective guard rail on the left side of the bed and the bottom of the bed. My plan is to bypass the alarm on the bed that goes off when the rail is moved. Once I arrive at that in-between space, which is my exit from bed, I continue scooting until I push my feet and legs through my exit. Just when I think I'm free and clear, I'm

## Two Days Before I'm Discharged

startled by a high-pitched sound, "beep, beep, beep . . ." that fills my room and the hallway. I freeze. *Ah crap!*, I think. A nurse in the room across the hall shouts, "Ms. Smith, Get back in the bed! Get back in the bed!" But I'm not moving my body back into the bed. The speech therapists who is helping Mrs. Masai in the next bed, runs from behind the curtain separating our beds, "Ms. Smith, what are you doing?" "I need to go to the bathroom. I called some time ago, but nobody has come," I respond in utter frustration. *What's the big deal?!*, I think. The therapist yells to the nurse across the hall, "I'll accompany Ms. Smith to the bathroom." I didn't know that the therapist was in the room, but I'm grateful she is. In the end, my mission is accomplished—with what seems to me as unnecessary hoopla.

Two days before I'm discharged, I need to use the bathroom, but the person in the room next door is using our bathroom. When I call for help to go to the bathroom, Keisha arrives and tells me she is taking me to another bathroom. She puts the belt around my waist and, holding the strip on the belt, she walks behind me. This is the first time that I'm walking with the therapy belt the distance from my room to the bathroom around the corner and down the hall, the same bathroom where Georgia treated me to a warm shower. As I walk, I'm looking down at my feet, which is what I was taught to do to maintain my balance. When I become distracted by my surroundings (e.g., the pictures on the wall, people in the hallway), I lose my balance. Although I'm looking down, watching where I place my feet, I can also see Dr. Milton and his entourage exit a patient's room just ahead of me. I can tell that Dr. Milton is surprised to see me walking; he has not seen me walk since I've been in the hospital. The chart in my room is seldom updated to show progress, I notice. Although I'm looking down to make sure that, with each step, I plant my feet properly on the ground, I can see that Dr. Milton is walking backwards behind Dr. Justin and the intern, observing how I'm walking. My mother taught us that we should see everything in a room when we enter it. In other words, we should always be consciously observant of our surroundings, not just what's directly in front of us, but the entire room. After a few seconds, Dr. Milton faces forward and rejoins his entourage as they continue their morning rounds and enter the next patient's room. I continue into the bathroom to my left.

Once I'm settled on the toilet, Keisha says, "Call me when you are ready [by pushing the help button], and I'll come back to get you." She is called away to help another patient. When I finish, I press the help button, and a very alarmed nurse answers, "What are you doing in there? How did you get there? Have you fallen?" Before I know it, three nurses descend on me in the bathroom. You'd have thought the bathroom was on fire with me in it! Innocent and wide-eyed, I explain. "Keisha brought me down here because somebody's in my bathroom. She told me to call for help, and she'd come back for me." That bathroom trip created a lot of unexpected excitement. I had no idea! That was both startling and exhilarating! A nurse accompanies me to my room, and I'm smiling the entire way back. She doesn't even have to hold my belt as I walk. I feel like the Energizer Bunny.

## 43

# Discharge from ERH

SINA HAS TO WORK so my discharge is delayed a day. Early Thursday morning, the day I was originally supposed to be discharged, Dr. Milton pops into my room.

"You are walking out of here soon!"

"Yes, I am."

"You have any questions?" he asks.

"No. . . . Oh, can I fly?"

"Of course you can fly. Where are you going?"

"To a [Wabash] creative writing retreat in North Carolina."

"Where in North Carolina?"

"I can't recall."

"Any more questions?"

"No."

"I look forward to seeing you walking out there somewhere," he says as he goes to check on Mrs. Masai.

I don't fly. I don't attend the Wabash Creative Writing Roundtable in July 2023 for two reasons. First, I don't think I have the cognitive or physical stamina to sit or think for long stretches of time. I was right; I attend the retreat the following year in 2024. Two, I want to be more independent when I fly for the first time after my stroke. I want to walk through the airport.

I'm glad to be going home, and I'm afraid. Despite the wonderful progress I've made, I have a long journey ahead of me. I'm lucky that my health insurance covers the overwhelming majority of my medical bills. I'm lucky that it pays for thirteen weeks of outpatient therapy beginning a week after my discharge. Most people don't have this kind of coverage. My mother never did; my sisters don't.

On the evening of Thursday, June 14, Sina drives nine hours from Columbus, directly to ERH in time for my 9:00 AM discharge process (actually, she's early). Sina is a skilled long-distance driver; she used to drive for Greyhound. The purpose of the informational meetings with speech, occupational, and physical therapists is to discuss my condition, progress, and needs, and to answer any questions we may have. Sina is in the waiting room at the end of the hall, I'm told. Accompanied by my speech therapist, I walk slowly down to meet her. I haven't seen her in over a year, I believe. I'm very emotional when I see her. Tears well up in my eyes, and she hugs me gently. I'm really happy to see Sina.

My colleague Raj arrives early too, and he carries most of my belongings to Sina's rental car after she hands him the car keys. When he returns, the nurse is going over my medications. Raj offers to pick up my prescriptions at CVS.

I remember two things from those informational meetings with the therapists, both from our time with Michael. First, Michael advises, "You are not supposed to cook!" He doesn't say, but I think he means that I shouldn't try to use a knife to chop up food, considering the weak condition of my hands. Or I shouldn't come close to fire given the numbness in my fingers. Don't know why I don't ask for clarification. It's probably because I know I'll cook when I'm ready. Right now, it's the last thing on my mind. Second, Michael makes the mistake of calling my sister "sweetheart." Sina corrects him, "My name is Jamesina." He probably couldn't remember the name "Jamesina," but he certainly didn't call her "sweetheart" again.

After we've had our meetings with the therapists, I leave ERH in a wheelchair. It's not my wheelchair. Quite reluctantly, I have ordered a wheelchair; the deductible alone was $350. I have resisted getting a wheelchair, not because of the cost, although it did give me pause. I don't want to become dependent on a wheelchair. *I'm afraid that I'll end up like my mother.* The speech therapist is more successful than Stacey, the physical therapist, in convincing me to purchase a wheelchair for use at home.

"You should get the wheelchair, just in case you need it."

*That's a lot of money for just in case*, I'm thinking. *They're just trying to sell me something.*

"You might need it if you go out somewhere in public."

"I don't see myself going out in public until I can walk longer distances."

"It won't hurt to have it, even if you don't use it. You never know."

"That's a good point."

Once home, I never go out anywhere in public where I need to use the wheelchair. But it does come in handy for months after my discharge, since I cannot stand for more than five to ten minutes without fatigue to brush my teeth, wash my face and body, and comb my hair. We set the wheelchair in front of the sink in the downstairs bathroom. I sit in it every day for at least an hour. The speech therapist was right about *just in case*.

Part 4

# Home and Nineteen Months Later

"We want a healthcare system that's available, affordable, accessible, and crisis responsive. It needs to be patient oriented. . . . We must educate, educate, educate. [We can't] continue to brag about the fact that we have the greatest sick-care system in the world [as opposed to a healthcare system]." —Dr. Jocelyn Elders, former Surgeon General[1]

---

1. Jocelyn Elders, Speech. In 1953, Elders joined the army as part of the Women's Medical Corp during the Korean War. As an army officer, she served as a trained physical therapist for injured soldiers. She is licensed pediatrician who also earned a degree in biochemistry in 1967 and became a full professor of pediatrics at the University of Arkansas in 1976.

## 44

# My Help Cometh from Sina!

I AM RELIEVED TO be home and determined to regain my "independence," but I'm also scared. I'm scared that my hopes are too big. I'm afraid because my sister, Sina, can only stay with me for about ten days. Then I'll be on my own. I fear that the physical therapists who told me that I should be good by the end of August are wrong. I'm afraid that the challenges I face will prove daunting. I'm afraid because my risk of having another stroke is greater now than before the stroke. I fear that life is passing me by. It frightens me that I may not be well enough to return to work in January 2024, teaching in the classroom and attending meetings, when the portion of my sick leave that covers 100 percent of my salary runs out. I can only live one day at a time. I have no choice. I had no choice before the stroke. But now I must also attend to the civil war in my body. I must give it my undivided attention. I cannot multitask my way out of it or through it.

CTS, my employer, owns the houses in which the majority of the faculty reside. After asking me what I need to prepare the house for my discharge, Dean Yoder ensures that the school installs safety bars in the downstairs bathroom. Sina and I order an easy-to-install railing to place around the downstairs toilet so that I have bars on both sides to hold onto to help myself on and off the toilet. Sina places the wheelchair in the bathroom so that I can sit in it when I'm brushing my teeth, washing my hands, combing my hair (which I cannot yet do), and bathing myself from the sink. Since walking up and down the two flights of stairs to my bedroom on the second floor is too difficult or strenuous, Sina brings the very sturdy blow-up mattress bed from upstairs, positions it in front of the sofa, plugs it in, flips the switch to inflate it, and place sheets and a blanket over it so that I can sleep downstairs. The living room is my bedroom for the next four to six months. It is also where I receive guests who bring dishes of food or visit with me. I sleep a lot; my body and my brain crave sleep.

Unfortunately, sleep is a privilege not everyone enjoys equally. Poverty impacts our quantity and quality of sleep. While the average person sleeps almost 300,000 hours during a lifetime, or one-third of their life, this number is significantly less for people living in poverty. Of people living below the poverty line, 33.6 percent get less than the recommended seven hours of sleep per night. According to data collected by the Center for Disease Control (CDC), "sleep may be affecting [our] health and wealth," and this is especially the case for people living below the poverty line,[1] not to mention those at or near the line. Emily Orminski argues that

> the sleep gap is a cyclical problem. Where you live is an ultimate social determinant of health. Thanks to redlining, gentrification, and other forces that drive financial insecurity, poor people are highly concentrated in areas with poor health outcomes. The common phrase "your zip code is more important than your genetic code" holds true for sleep cycles as well. Both racial minorities and low-income individuals often reside in communities where many factors play into their lack of sleep and sleep quality. Low-income people are most likely to work more than one job to make ends meet, which directly affects the amount of time they have to sleep. They are also more likely to live in areas with more air, light and noise pollution, and in food deserts, a large contributor to poor diets and food insecurity.... Those experiencing poverty are also relegated to areas with high levels of toxic stress, adding to the stress from lower-paying jobs, systemic racism and financial insecurity. These social and environmental factors all work hand in hand to reduce both the amount as well as the quality of sleep.[2]

For African Americans, this sleep deprivation goes back to enslavement, when the enslaved were required to stay awake so that they could be ready to provide for every need, demand, or whim of the enslaver or slave master, from sunup to sundown. Falling asleep was the most common

---

1. Orminski, "Sleep Is a Cyclical Inequity for Those in Poverty."
2. Orminski, "Sleep Is a Cyclical Inequity for Those in Poverty."

transgression for which the enslaved were punished. They lived toturesome lives; sleep deprivation is torture.[3]

My post-stroke body demands more sleep. So did my pre-stroke body. Sleep is one of the first things we do after my bed and the bathroom are set up. I fall asleep. Sina takes a nap. As I said, she came straight to the hospital after her nine-hour drive from Columbus. After her long nap, the second thing Sina does for me is run a warm bath. I have not had a bath in a bathtub since before my stroke. Words cannot express how I feel sinking down into the hot, soapy water. I linger. I don't yet realize how difficult it will be for Sina to get me out of the bathtub. My feet are more useless than I thought. Sina lets the water out of the tub before placing a towel over my body. While she is lifting me out of the tub, I'm triaging. I'm trying to keep the towel in place so as not to bare my naked body to my sister and the air, but her focus is getting me out of the tub without dropping me. "This ain't the time for that. We need to get you out of the tub!" I release my pride, and the towel follows. With her arms under my armpits and quite a bit of effort, Sina lifts and drags me out of the tub. I couldn't help her. Clearly, we won't be doing that again during her short stay. Sina purchases rubber bath mats for both bathrooms, upstairs and downstairs. Until I am strong enough, I wash my body from the bathroom sink. I shower only once a week until I am stronger. I am weak, and I look frail.

---

3. See Smith, *Insights from African American Interpretation*, chapter 4.

# 45

# Meal Train, DoorDash, and Chicken Soup

CHRISTINE YODER AND LISA Weaver set up a meal train schedule for me. Many of my colleagues at CTS sign up to prepare and bring home-cooked and restaurant-prepared meals and donated gift cards to DoorDash for Sina and me during my first few weeks at home. Sina also cooks a few meals herself and we order food through DoorDash using the gift cards. I didn't know the culinary skills my colleagues possessed. The homemade chicken soup Christine Yoder brings on one visit is wonderful! A former student, Leo Allen, comes by to visit and offers to cook. I caution him not to neglect his studies but I am appreciative that he offers to cook a few meals for me (e.g., homemade chili), and I reimburse him for the food purchased. He refuses to accept any additional payment for his effort. Other colleagues who bring food and stay a while to visit with me include Dr. Brennan Breed and his wife, Catherine. Brennan makes the most flavorful grilled chicken I've ever tasted. And Catherine's homemade pesto is excellent. Sina and I happily eat the grilled chicken and pesto for days. Dr. Raj Nadella makes homemade dahl (white lentil soup) and rice—heavenly. Raj's wife, Amy, brings the food to me, and we sit and talk for quite awhile. We weep and hug each other just before she leaves. I am so grateful for Amy's vulnerability and authenticity. Abby Myers, Jake's wife, makes some mean vegan meals. I am grateful for their friendship and generosity during my first few weeks home and beyond.

## Meal Train, DoorDash, and Chicken Soup

As much as I dearly appreciate the food that colleagues, students, and/or friends donate to me during the crucial days of my home recovery, they often cook too much food. It will be a while yet before I can eat the amount of food that I ate before the stroke. Every mealtime, Sina fixes a plate of food for me, I walk the few feet from my bed in the living room to sit at the dining table, eat a few bites, and I feel so full that my body cannot tolerate more. I tell Sina, "Wrap it up, please" or "Leave it there on the table, I'll be back to eat the rest." I never make it back to the table; Sina ends up eating the food herself or tossing what I have left after it remains in the fridge too long. I really try each time to eat more, but I feel like I have failed. Sina assures me, "You're doing okay. You're eating fine." I'm grateful for her response. Otherwise, I might have been even more anxious about not yet being able to eat as I normally would.

# 46

# "Is this the hardest thing you've ever done?"

I'M APPRECIATIVE OF THE friends and colleagues who visit me in my home while I sit or lie on the makeshift bed in the living room and who spend considerable time to be present with me. One of them is Lavonne Rennick. We grew up together in the projects in Columbus, Ohio; attended Central High School together; and have spent time together since I moved to Georgia almost six years ago. Lavonne checks on me and drops by a couple of times after work, before her body summons her to attend to her own health issues. Dr. Ericka Dunbar, an African American Hebrew Bible/Old Testament scholar and colleague, stops in; she brings me a beautiful floral arrangement. Ericka is an assistant professor at Baylor University in Waco, Texas, but she has a home in Atlanta with her husband. Christine Yoder drops in quite often to talk and check on my progress. Her father suffered a stroke about two years ago and is recovering well. Dr. Renita Weems is originally from Atlanta, with family still here. Renita is the first (she says the second) Black woman to earn a PhD in Hebrew Bible/Old Testament and a public theologian, colleague, and friend. I'm so happy that she stops by for about an hour to see about me. She pointedly asks, "Is this the hardest thing you've ever done?" "Yes, this is the hardest thing I've ever done," I solemnly reply.

# 47

# Outpatient Therapy

On June 22, 2023, I start outpatient therapy at Emory Brain Health Center (EBHC), a week after ERH discharges me to go home. I attend three days each week. I meet for forty-five minutes each with the speech, occupational, and physical therapists. I'm released from outpatient therapy on September 28, 2023.

My first two weeks are rough. Physically, I'm still weak and frail. The occupational therapists work primarily with my right hand. I cooperate. I feel that my right hand will improve as it heals. Of course, I do the exercises, and I use my hand when I do the routine tasks that I'm capable of when at home. I wring out my washcloth and eat with my left hand. I don't let my right hand just hang by my side, as the occupational therapist accuses me of doing. I purchase a hand grip and multicolored stiff foam cubes, which I pick up with my right hand and place in a basket. It's important that we know our own bodies and that we don't allow others to limit our capabilities.

The primary occupational therapist, Ashley, a white woman, recorded the following in her after visit notes on my last day of outpatient therapy: "Continues to demonstrate poor ROM [range of motion] of R [right] index finger, not allowing her to perform a tip-to-tip pinch. Edema continues to persist in the thumb, index and middle digit of her RUE [right upper extremity] as well." Ashley works on my right hand and particularly my right index finger a lot. While therapists know what they know, they do not know a patient's body as well as the patient knows her own body. At one point, Ashley tells me that if I don't bend my right index finger during therapy, she is afraid it will remain as it is. One day Ashley is so frustrated with me and my finger that she yells, "Bend that finger!" Everyone in the therapy room turns to look at me (or her). I am angry and hurt. But as a Black woman with a medical disability, I dare not yell back; I will be viewed as the problem. I remember thinking, *There are people in this room in worse shape than I am. I have not heard one therapist yell at a patient before Ashley yells at me. Is she racist? Or is there another reason she would yell at me in particular?* Ashley can tell that I am visibly upset; I don't hide my anger or pain. I don't remember what exactly I eventually said to her or how long it took me to say it. At one point, Ashley does apologize, "I'm not trying to hurt you intentionally. I know you are doing your best." I'm thinking, *So, then, why the need to yell, if you know I'm doing my best?!* It wouldn't be the last time I must address the callousness I feel Ashley demonstrates toward my inability to bend my right index finger. She sometimes forces my fingers closed to make a fist. She does it slowly but forces it beyond my comfort. Yet, as I eventually express to the Indian Asian woman therapist who works under Ashley's supervision and follows her instructions when Ashley is absent, "I thought you all told us not to inflict pain upon ourselves. Then, why do you think it's okay for you to do so?!"

In the US, there are few Black physical therapists relative to white therapists and in proportion to the Black population; this is a general problem in the medical professions. According to Avery Simmons, "In 2021, only 5% of physical therapists were Black, while 78% were white. In contrast, the population of the United States is 12% Black or African American, and only 58% white (non-Hispanic).... [H]aving Black medical professionals leads to better care for Black people."[1] There's also the problem of white myths about Black pain. According to Janice Sabin, 50 percent of "white medical trainees believe such myths as black people have thicker skin or less sensitive nerve endings than white people."[2] Such myths have a long history going back at least to the father of modern gynecology, Dr. J. Marion Sims, who operated on Black teenage girls without the use of anesthesia.

One of the things that Beth, the physical therapist, works with me to improve is balance. I have very little balance. I attach a copy of a balance exercise sheet under a magnet on my fridge door. Every time I go to the fridge, I stop and practice the balance exercises. Right foot back, left foot

---

1. Simmons, "Why We Need More Black Physical Therapists."
2. Sabin, "How We Fail Black Patients in Pain."

back, right foot forward . . . I do it as quickly as I can each time. The pace at which I go through the entire sheet improves, as does my balance.

After eight weeks of outpatient therapy, I can lift the two-pound free weights, walk forward and backward on the treadmill for a total of ten minutes, ride the stationary bike for ten minutes, and walk up and down the back steps once, to name a few of my achievements. Today, I can lift my twenty-five-pound free weight and twelve-pound weighted ball; walk an hour on my treadmill, including twenty minutes on incline; walk 6,000 to 10,000 steps outdoors; and run up and down the steps from the first to the second floor at home.

For the first week of therapy, Sina drives me and sits with me for the initial assessment. I am still quite frail and very weak. Sometimes Marcia Riggs, Sharon Ozonuwe (who visits from New Jersey), Napria (who arrives and stays a week), or Samatha drives me to EBHC. Having to depend on other people for rides to therapy for eight weeks, three times per week, is a lot. By week six, I call an Uber. By the end of that week, I ask the occupational therapist about the certification that stroke survivors are supposed to obtain before driving again. She says that she can and will do it for me; she never mentions it again. I ask my primary care doctor to send a referral to ERH for their certification; she does, but I never receive a response. Weeks seven and eight, I drive my car to EBHC anyway. It's like riding a bike—well, almost. A couple of years before my stroke, Genetta Hatcher, Eva Melton, and I went on a girl's trip to Florida where we rode bikes for the first time since who knows when (at least that was the case for me); I fell off the bike three times. I had on a helmet. Didn't hurt myself! It tickled me; I laughed after each tumble. Thank God, when I push the button to start my Honda Civic, it tells the driver in red letters which pedal is the brake and which is the gas. After that, I'm fine.

In week eight, I can walk six laps around the path from the hallway that stretches out in front of the door of the therapy room and up to the waiting area, right turn past the elevators on my right, right turn down the opposite hallway, and finally a right turn down the back hallway leading back to the therapy room door where we began. I complete the six laps in less than six minutes. When I began, I could barely make two laps in more than six minutes. And I couldn't do it without stumbling into the walls or stopping to rest. Regarding the stationary bike and the treadmill, I progressed from one minute to ten minutes.

Speech therapy helped me to realize how much my post-stroke brain needs "to-do lists." If I do not prepare a "to-do list" *and* remember that I have a "to-do list," I forget my "to-do's" and appointments. Simply putting items on my iPhone calendar, as I did before my stroke, does not work. I must write out a list on paper, the old-fashioned way, and keep that list where I can see it all day—on the kitchen table.

# Outpatient Therapy

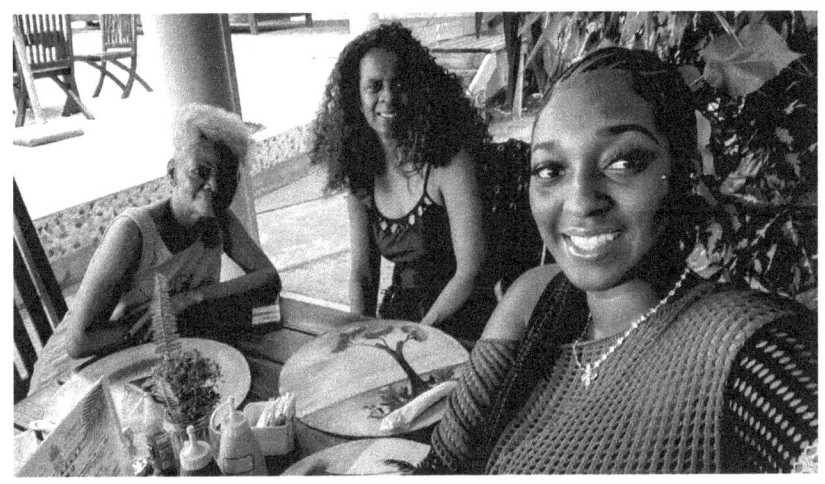

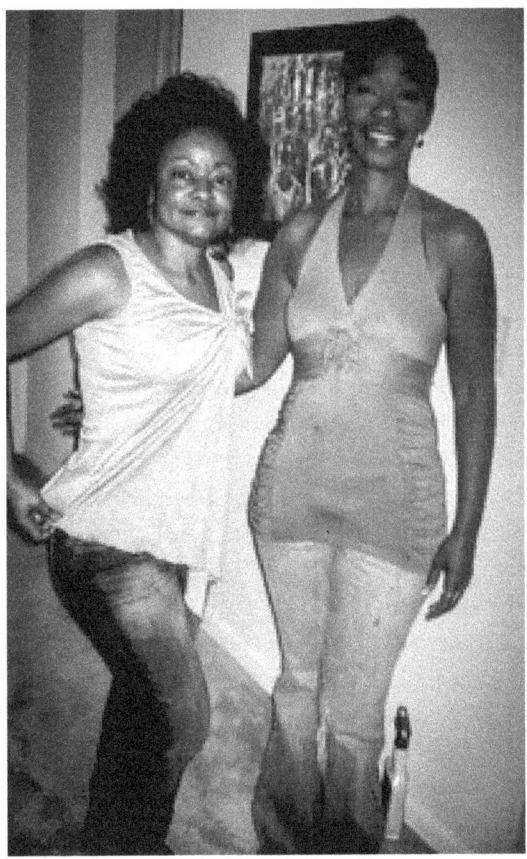

# 48

# Back in the Classroom

My health insurance allows for twelve weeks of fully paid sick leave; after that I would have to live on 60 percent of my salary. I have prayed and worked toward the goal of returning to the classroom, and I do so in J-term of January 2024. The first class that I teach seven months after my stroke is an advanced-level, weeklong intensive entitled "Womanist and Feminist Interpretation and Justice." The course participants are a small, diverse group of students in either the doctor of ministry or master of theological studies programs. Three of the students are African Americans (comprising a cisgender male pastor, a trans woman, and a cisgender woman), one is an Asian American (South Korean) woman, and one a white male with an earned PhD in history from the country of Georgia. The students are required to lead discussion of several assigned readings and raise questions for discussion. I'm generally pleased with the manner in which they engage the various voices in the reading materials and one another, as well as the questions they raise.

Toward the end of the course, I treat the students to lunch at a Korean BBQ restaurant in Decatur. It is not my first time at a Korean BBQ restaurant. The Korean Biblical Colloquium (KBC), which meets at the annual Society of Biblical Literature (SBL) conference, invites me from time to time as a panelist in their sessions. Whenever I attend KBC, my South Korean friends and colleagues treat me afterwards to their annual community meal at a local Korean BBQ wherever the SBL meeting is convened (e.g., San Diego, Denver, Boston, Chicago). Six months after my stroke in

## Back in the Classroom

November 2023, I serve on a KBC panel as a respondent to Cathy Park Hong's book *Minor Feelings: An Asian American Reckoning*. I'm especially intrigued by her chapter on bad English. Hong writes that bad English:

> was once a source of shame but now I say it proudly: bad English is my heritage. I share a literary lineage with writers who make unmastering English their rallying cry—who queer it, twerk it, hack it, cannibalize it, other it by hijacking English and warping it to a fugitive tongue. To other English is to make audible the imperial power sown into the language, to slit English open so it's dark histories slide out.[1]

The work of Black linguists like Geneva Smitherman and John McWhorter, as well as Hong's book, encourage me to rethink the notion of proper English in relation to student engagement and grading. What we consider major is perhaps minor. For Hong, minor feelings are neither insignificant nor harmless.

At the Korean BBQ in Decatur, diverse slim cuts of well-seasoned meats—chicken, beef, pork, and shrimp—are cooked on a hot steel surface that is fired underneath and sits in the middle of the table. Small dishes containing several different sauces, as well as kimchi, white rice, and salads, are placed on the table. For one price, you can eat all you can hold. So good!

Having a meal with family, friends, colleagues or even strangers is not a minor thing. Evidently, there's an app called "Diner" that brings strangers together for a meal; its intention is to disrupt the pervasive loneliness that so many people are experiencing. While we are at the Korean BBQ, my Korean American woman student comes to life! And she brings that energy into our final few course sessions. At the restaurant, she guides us through the menu, telling us what's what, and she takes over the ordering process. Sister even turns the meat as it cooks and passes it around the table. Before this moment, she had been virtually silent throughout the course. It's a minor thing; but it's major!

---

1. Hong, *Minor Feelings*, 97.

# 49

# Palimpsest

A SCAR ON THE pinky finger of my right hand that resulted from a wound I suffered after shutting it in a car door is barely recognizable. A man had given me a ride home from the bus stop, a distance of about two miles; most times I walked the distance. When I realized my finger was caught in the car door, I quickly opened it to release my finger before the car drove off. Funny thing, my embarrassment at shutting my own finger in a man's car door was like Motrin for my excruciating pain. I didn't cry until I got into the apartment. As soon as I crossed the threshold and shut the door, I screamed and cried "bloody murder."

Only recently, on October 26, 2024, about sixteen months after my stroke, I notice that the scar on my right-hand pinky finger has faded. I am massaging it with Shea butter when I notice. I've known that scar since I was eighteen years old, shortly after I graduated from high school. On that same pinky finger is a recent scar that darkens my skin; it's collateral damage from the stroke and it resulted from resting my eating utensils on that part of my finger before I could remember how to hold them the way I did before the stroke. The old scar has benefited from the consistent therapeutic attention I give to the new scar. Sometimes, decades-old scars vanish as we nurse new scars. It's similar to a palimpsest, where recent writing effaces the old, making room for the new, but traces of the old remain visible, even if barely. Traces of the older scar on my pinky finger are mostly imprinted only in my memory and no longer in my flesh.

Reflecting on the incident of shutting my finger in a car door, it is the first time I remember that I *have* been in the ER before as a patient. My stroke was not the first medical emergency that sent me to the ER, but it is the third and the most serious, and also potentially fatal. The second ER visit involved a car door too. I must have been a magnet for car doors, as are the tires on my car for Georgia nails. I don't recall how old I was, but it happened over twenty years ago. I returned a vehicle to a car rental agency at Port Columbus airport. In a hurry, I either opened or closed my driver's side door too quickly before my head cleared the top edge of the door, and I smacked myself in the face with the door, leaving a gash just below my right eyebrow. For the first time in my life, I received stitches; the scar completely healed and disappeared some years ago.

# 50

# Facebook Updates
## Stroke Recovery Progress

THE THERAPISTS TOLD ME that the most rapid progress takes place within the first year after the stroke. After that, recovery continues, but it's slower. I also read somewhere that the extremities, which are farthest from the heart or the brain, are the last to heal. Sometimes, I post stroke recovery updates on my Facebook page. I've also joined a number of stroke recovery groups, including Stroke Sisters, Stroke Warrior Recovery Exercise With Mind Set Up, and Fitness After Stroke: A Stroke Buddies Group, where stroke survivors encourage one another and share information and advice. During my first year post-stroke, I can't type using my right hand, but I discover the microphone on my iPhone and dictate my posts. Why hadn't I noticed that function before now?! It would have made life so much easier. As Dr. Renita Weems says, "The teacher appears when the student shows up." The following posts are from September 22, 2023, to December 27, 2024, which spans a year and seven months post-stroke.

### September 22, 2023

I remain thankful for your prayers, words of encouragement, and gifts. Last week my physical therapist said that she's confident that I can go into any store now since I was able to walk for six minutes straight without stopping and at a pretty fast pace, going faster than I have been able to do at this point. This week I walked 3,000 steps in the neighborhood and only rested once. Today I went into the farmers' market for the first time since I've been sick, to pick up a few things. My speech therapist, who has been working with me to make sure I am at my base in terms of my higher-level thinking, discharged me on Tuesday. While I am not eager to read academic books, I am reading a little. I did, however, spend an hour tutoring two Greek students this week at my home; I enjoyed it. I will work with my physical therapist one more week and with my occupational therapist two more weeks. Some healing can only come as my body heals, which can take time, and other healing flows from doing certain exercises repeatedly. I am having no problems driving my car as necessary.

## October 8, 2023

Update #strokerecovery: I am deeply grateful for the prayers, encouraging words, meals with colleagues, and gifts that I have received since and before my last update. I received text messages, phone calls, emails, flowers, a case of Ensure, a fruit and nut box, an excellent free yoga class, and so on. On Tuesday of this past week, I was released from outpatient therapy. Now it is up to me to continue the exercises and techniques I learned. I am now sleeping upstairs in my own bed because I can now navigate the stairs so well 😌. I am cooking most of my own meals. I went to the farmers' market for the very first time and very slowly carried four bags back to my car 😋. I snapped some fresh green beans and cooked them. I decided this morning that I'm not going to obsess about gaining weight. As long as I am eating healthy and all my body functions are good. I don't want to eat ice cream to gain weight; I don't want to eat a lot of unhealthy sweets and unhealthy things that I had stopped eating. I have less pain in my feet and the right hand. I still have the numbness, swelling, and burning sensation, but I'll take that over the pain I had. I must continue to allow my body to heal at its own pace, while doing my part. I am thankful to be alive and to have hope for the future. I am thinking quite a lot about the ways in which I want my life to be different and what I will do to make it happen.

## October 27, 2023

Update #stroke-recovery: I continue to be thankful for your prayers, texts, emails, and gifts. My stamina continues to improve. I had a first (and hopefully last) fall in the house; turned too fast, tripped over my feet, and went down on the floor; scared me more than anything. Escaped with a minor scratch and a bruise or two. Balance is something I continue to work on. As I go about daily living, I see improvement. The first time I washed my hair after arriving home from the hospital, I could barely tolerate lifting my arms over my head to put rollers in the top of my hair. It would take me about an hour. Today it took me about fifteen minutes and my arms were not very tired. This past Sunday I walked over 4,000 steps, which is the most that I have walked outside since being home. This week I walked for thirty minutes on the treadmill (twice) at a moderate pace. I am sleeping good without the aid of Tylenol PM or pain. I still experience quite a bit of fatigue; some of it may be attributable to medication. The doctor decreased the dosage of one of my high blood pressure medications at my request, since my numbers are very good. I'm hoping I can come off of that particular medication in the coming months. So this is all good news for the most part. Please keep your prayers coming as well as your positive thoughts. Thank you so much and take care of yourselves.

PS: when I told my older sister about the fall, she said, "Mitzi, you didn't have that far to fall." 😁

## November 5, 2023

Tomorrow, November 6, is my birthday. On May 24 of this year, I wasn't sure that I would see another birthday on this earth. It was on that day that I entered the ER at Emory Hospital and spent three or four days in the ICU until they stabilized my blood pressure. It was a surreal experience. At first I didn't know if I would survive. Eventually, I realized that my disposition, my attitude, would determine my survival. This has been the hardest thing I have ever had to do. I had never even been admitted to a hospital before, but I spent about four weeks between the hospital and the rehab hospital. In the past five months I have gone from not being able to walk to walking more than 4,000 steps and thirty minutes on a treadmill. I have progressed from not being able to stand on my feet for five to ten minutes to standing on my feet for an hour or more. I want to make each day count as I continue to recover but I must remember that each day is a day of recovery. The most rapid recovery takes place within a year of stroke; it's only been five months for me. I am truly thankful for every single prayer, kind word, gift (small or large), meal, and help. I am grateful to the doctors, nurses, custodians, therapists, family members, colleagues, and friends who contributed to my recovery. I am grateful for a second chance at life and plan to make the most of it. Happy birthday to me.

## November 8, 2023

Today, Tina Pippin and I walked a mile and a half around Avondale Lake. It's 81 degrees in Georgia.

## November 13, 2023

Today, I clipped my own toenails using my left hand. First time since stroke. Who knows, maybe I'll be left-handed or ambidextrous when I fully recover 😀!

PS: the last time I went to the nail salon to have my toenails and fingernails clipped, there were several older gentlemen in the salon getting their toenails clipped. The manicurist asked one of the men why his wife was not there. He said he came alone because she has to go out of town. His wife told him, "Put your big boy pants on and go by yourself." LOL.

## November 17, 2023

Taking my first flight since my stroke to AAR/SBL. Lyft driver got me to airport in record time. He drove like he was in the Indy 500. "God, don't let me go like this after surviving a stroke."

Took my time walking through airport. Proud of myself. Safe travels everyone.

## November 18, 2023

Yesterday, I walked about 7,000 steps. I overwalked my feet. Yes, that is a thing now. By about 4:00 PM I was in bed in my hotel room here in San Antonio, Texas. I had breakfast in my hotel room and now I'm going to write my response/presentation for a 4:00 PM book review panel with Joseph Marchal, NaShieka Knight, and Angela Parker. I am grateful for their critical engagement with my new book *Chloe and Her People*. I've got to work with my body and not against it. I and my body are on the same side of this internal war. I am grateful for the hugs and conversations with friends and colleagues yesterday.

## January 1, 2024

I decide that I am strong enough to get out of the bathtub on my own using my hands and feet. I did it! I am grateful. From now on I take at least one warm bath a week.

## April 28, 2024

I'm also back to using the free weights I used pre-stroke. I can swing the twenty-pound kettle bell, lift the ten-pound weights in each hand to do shoulder presses, and so on. I'm determined as much as possible to be back and better. Women need strength training and weight-bearing exercises like squats, especially as we age (like wine).

## April 28, 2024

My mother, Flora Smith, didn't have the health insurance that I have (she had zip, nada, until she became unable to walk at all and then received Medicaid, which was better but grossly insufficient); was less likely than me to find a doctor who cared and treated her with compassion; never had sick leave; and suffered from too many illnesses starting in early childhood. Yet she never expressed hopelessness, refused to be limited by her traumas, and wouldn't let me sulk for too long. I wish she had better; it pains me to even think about it. I have so much more starting with what she planted in me. I can be temporarily sad, down, depressed but I cannot choose defeat.

## June 17, 2024

Comedian Keith Robinson's [stroke survivor] show "Different Strokes" is HILARIOUS!

## September 4, 2024

About two weeks ago I finished my first academic essay (other than two short forewords) since my stroke. A wonderful accomplishment, especially since I didn't want to read anything until about January of this year and then didn't want to focus on heavy academic work. The essay I wrote will be published as a chapter in my Luke book and in a book on parables. It is a rereading of Luke's slave parables. Now working to finish another essay and then back to Luke, my stroke memoir, and *OUP* [Oxford University Press] *Handbook*. Don't worry, since I'm on study leave I'm still getting the rest my body requires as I continue my stroke recovery.

## October 15, 2024

I have a book contract for my stroke memoir. Working title: *Not Wanting a Thing to Be the Thing*. #CascadeBooks

## September 6, 2024

I'm about fifteen months post-stroke. Does anyone else experience unusual bruising after leg stretching exercises? My doc says my platelets are better; not disconcertingly low. Took baby aspirin prior to stroke and no problem. But I'm going to change to every other day for a while to see if it impacts the situation.

[Posted in the Fitness after Stroke: A Stroke Buddies Group. Two people respond with the same issue; only one is taking baby aspirin.]

## September 16, 2024

I'm not sure at what point after my stroke this started, but my nose runs every time I eat, as if I'm always eating hot, spicy food. Is this happening for anyone else?

## September 29, 2024

Good morning! I now have enough sensory feeling and dexterity in my thumb and the first two fingers of my right hand to put my hoop earrings into my ear lobes and without looking in the mirror. Progress! I exercise, stretch, bend, massage my fingers and hands a lot when I'm awake. Next goal is to be able to put post earrings in. I'm beginning to pick up small objects with the fingers on my right hand.

## November 3, 2024

I purchased the gold-coated bracelet yesterday at the mall with my cousin Tiffany. I had been contemplating for some time an inspirational bracelet. This fits what I need, almost a year and a half post-stroke. The amethyst is my mother's birth stone and I'm a womanist. Live as if #TheBestIsYetToCome.

## November 20, 2024

Did your stroke impact your kidneys? To what extent?

[Posted in Stroke Sisters Facebook group. One member said it did impact her kidneys. Another replied "I had issues with my kidney Shrinking due to lack of oxygen from FMD. After the stroke had more imaging, guess what?! Kidney back to normal size and appearance and my renal arteries were patent. Totally miraculous." Most said "No."]

## December 27, 2024

Last night I braided the hair on the top of my head into one plait using both hands. Thumb and two fingers still numb and partially stiff but agility is returning. Elated! Force yourself to use it or it will gladly lay dormant.

# 51

# Kidney Disease?!

I don't know that the stroke has negatively impacted my kidneys until I have a series of blood tests taken by my primary care doctor. She refers me to a nephrologist, a kidney specialist. I didn't know until recently that the word *nephron* means kidney! I learned that term in November 2024 from a doctor's Instagram post testing users on their knowledge of medical terminology. I got a few of them correct but soon grew frustrated with him. *Just tell us what they mean!*

According to the National Kidney Foundation, "33% of U.S. adults are at risk for kidney disease. Minorities face higher risk due to diabetes and high blood pressure." Obesity, heart disease, and perhaps health care also place minorities at greater risk for kidney disease. The famous African American anti-lynching activist, journalist, and abolitionist, Ida B. Wells, died of kidney disease in 1931. On July 4, 2003, the African American bass crooner Barry White died of kidney failure, hypertension, adult-onset diabetes, and finally a stroke as he awaited a kidney transplant. Stevie Wonder underwent a successful kidney transplant in 2019.

My primary care doctor recommends a particular nephrologist, but I decide to stay within the Emory system. Access to my medical records is a necessity. Some doctors know they have access to MyChart online but fail to use it for whatever reason. My mother had many doctors who didn't know her history because records were not as available as they are now. Thank you, former President Obama. Obama signed laws to fast-track the adoption and meaningful use of digital medical records. Based on his years of expertise and very good patient reviews, I choose Dr. Harold Franch at Emory.

When I see Dr. Franch, the blood tests show that I have stage 3a chronic kidney disease as a result of the stroke. Kidney disease is scary stuff. I have a friend and colleague who was seeking a kidney donation at the time; as of today, December 24, she has had a kidney transplant from a donor who had died. When she was told that she had kidney disease, it was also stage 3a. Dr. Franch is encouraging; to put things in perspective, he reminds me, "You know people can live well with only one good functioning kidney." Based on many tests done on the many vials of blood they drained from my body, he sees no signs of progression with the disease, which is good. There's no protein in my blood. He advises, "The more vegetables you eat, the better."

I love vegetables. We grew up on vegetables. We couldn't afford meat. It seems the opposite today. Vegetables are expensive and not as accessible to all people in every place! Most of our diet growing up consisted of vegetables and legumes or beans. There's not a vegetable that I hate or won't eat raw or when it's seasoned and cooked properly. Okra, brussels sprouts, eggplant, carrots, cauliflower, greens. I'll eat them all and love it! My mother grew up on a farm where, of course, they ate lots of vegetables, as well as a variety of meats or flesh, from pig feet and ears to catfish. But we grew up in poverty and not on a farm. Our diet consisted of lots of beans, cornbread, and, when we could afford it, vegetables from the vegetable market or the truck that would come through the neighborhood. I think that is unheard of in poor neighborhoods today. When money was low (halfway through the month) and food scarce, Mommy sent us into the nearby fields to pick dandelion greens. Today, dandelion greens are sold at the local farmers' market at about $3 per measly bunch. You'd have to buy five to six bunches for a decent pot of greens. As the Netflix docuseries *You Are What You Eat: A Twin Experiment* shows, the quality of our food has rapidly deteriorated. Prices have skyrocketed. I don't know when I last ate any strawberries, oranges, or blueberries that didn't taste bitter. Despite that, I buy my fruits and vegetables primarily from the Dekalb farmers' market. Without reliable transportation, it is difficult or impossible to access most farmers' markets, since many are located primarily in suburban areas and a distance from public transportation. Dekalb is near public transportation. I'm proud that the farmers' market in Decatur takes the EBT cards for people who don't have cash or credit, but if you are like many Americans subsisting on credit

## Kidney Disease?!

cards, you're out of luck. They take no credit cards! So you are forced to pay the higher prices at big chain grocery stores, if you are fortunate enough to have one in your neighborhood. Only within this last decade or so, was a big chain supermarket built within the Detroit city limits. The thing is that food, good affordable food, is the best medicine for our bodies, and it has become inaccessible for too many people.

Lisa Weaver comes to visit me the week of November 19, 2024. She is in town to attend a friend's retirement celebration. I tell her that I have stage 3a chronic kidney disease. She seems more alarmed than I am. A renewed sense of dread overcomes me at about four in the morning. I reach for my phone, which I rarely do during the night anymore, and search for "best foods for chronic kidney diseases." My doctor could or should have said more than "eat plenty of vegetables." Damn, it seems I may be eating a lot of vegetables and fruit that are harmful to my condition, foods high in potassium. Every green is no longer my best friend! Dear God. As soon as I can that day, I go to the farmers' market. I buy arugula (been awhile) instead of spinach, expensive malnourished-looking cauliflower, brussels sprouts, sea bass steaks at $24 a pound, more blueberries (ran out), more shredded carrots, and eggs (but I'll no longer be eating the yolks)! Whew! I forgot the cabbage! I don't know if I dodged the bullet or if there was a bullet to dodge. I'll know when I see my nephrologist again.

## 52

# Fragments

### Fear

Post stroke, I fear being in crowds of people or in vulnerable spaces that require an ability to quickly evade danger. Anna Kendrick's 2023 Netflix film *Woman of the Hour* reminds us that women walk through a patriarchal, misogynistic world with a certain kind of justifiable fear. On October 15, 2024, the first day of early voting in general election in Georgia, I drive to the polling place nearest and most familiar to me. I plan to enthusiastically and without reservation cast my vote for Vice President Kamala Harris for President of the United States of America. It's about 9:00 AM, about an hour after I had a tire checked and replaced; the tire had a bubble in it. The polling place is crowded with a long line snaking around outside. While standing outside in the slowly moving line, I notice a Black man about forty or fiftyish and average height and appearance periodically staring. Whenever I look forward, he stares. I don't stare back. After about forty-five minutes, I finally move inside the polling place doors. The line is longer than I thought. I still have a ways to go before reaching the brave Black women poll workers—the Ruby Freemans and Shay Mosses—working the desk where we present our IDs. The man who keeps staring at me is ahead of me by about twenty people. After I proudly and optimistically cast my vote for Harris and the Democrats downballot, I exit the polling place and walk the distance between the polling place to my car in the crowded lot where people meander to and fro. People use the same lot to visit other state agencies in the complex. Given my short stature, it would be difficult to see me against that background. I arrive at my car. While getting my keys from my handbag, I notice a car approaching, which is not unusual or alarming in this busy context. The car stops; it could be stopping to yield the right of way to pedestrians and other vehicles. It lingers, and I look around. The man driving the stopped car is the same one who was staring at me in the voting line. My antennae are up.

"Are you married?"

I pause, thinking *Do I lie or tell the truth?* A woman should not have to lie to be safe.

"No, I'm not married." I continue unlocking my car door.

"Can I give you my card to call me?"

"No, I don't call strangers."

Luckily, the stranger respects my response and drives away. A man will call a woman a "whore" for saying "no." Women have been harmed and murdered for ignoring men's catcalls. Remember Caroline Nosal, Janese Talton-Jackson, Lisa and Anna Trubnikova, Lakeeya Walker, Raelynn Vincent, Andrea Farrington, Paris Shashay, Janese Talton-Jackson, and too many unknown women who are dead or seriously injured because they didn't respond to a man as he thought they should. Women are damned if they do, damned if they don't. The incident rattles me when I consider this man waited, watched, and followed me through the busy parking lot. That's unnerving.

As I recover, I wonder whether I'm fast enough or strong enough to escape and survive potentially dangerous situations. For this reason, I don't go too far by myself and certainly not at night. I was not a fan of enormous crowds before my stroke. Now I fear them.

## Walking

While in San Diego for our annual SBL meeting in late November 2024, I am amazed how fast I'm walking, speed-walking actually, between the Hilton Bayfront Hotel and the San Diego Convention Center. My legs and brain are in sync again as I walk quickly to avoid the cold wind and arrive at my sessions on time. When I don't walk daily, I experience a little regression. My muscles feel sluggish and need a warming-up period, which was not the case pre-stroke. Twenty months later that is improving. I also know when I've crossed the 6,000-step mark; my tailbone stiffens and is uncomfortable. I must sit for a few minutes and then I can resume. Walking with Dr. Tina Pippin, a few CTS students, and my former CTS colleague Dr. Haruko Ward around a nearby lake has been very helpful.

## Brain Health

Speaking of brain health, talking and walking can be a form of "dual-task" walking. According to NeuroLaunch, dual-tasking "involves performing a cognitive task while you walk, like reciting the alphabet backward or solving mental math problems. It's a great way to improve your cognitive flexibility and multitasking abilities. Just think of it as foot–brain connection . . . on steroids!"[1]

On December 5, 2024, I return to the Duolingo app to practice my Spanish language skills, which I abandoned when I had what I think was my first stroke prior to hospitalization for the third stroke. In the Duolingo review, I miss only two items, one by accidentally clicking the wrong answer, which happens often, given the numbness in my fingers. I decide to return to my lessons after a neurologist on Instagram says that one way to support brain health is to learn a new language. I'm working on consistency. "Learning is plasticity," according to the Master Class series "Brain Health." It's important to expose ourselves to new things, like new languages, driving routes, games, and so on. I'm now learning some Italian for a trip to Rome.

## Feet and Hands

Every now and then, I experience moments of panic and very short bouts of crying when I awake to the reality that my feet are still numb and the joints that connect my toes to my feet are stiff, the left less so than the right. I cannot spread the toes on my right foot. I cannot pose in "downward dog" unless I wear shoes to support my toes. Crossing my legs while lying down causes pains to shoot through my legs. My calves still cramp, not as often as they used to, but it's more painful when they do. The last time they cramped, I cried out while massaging them as deeply as I could. I panicked! But not for long. I think, *My feet are better than they used to be.* I have a

---

1. NeuroLaunch Editorial Team, "Walking Brain."

ways to go, but I've come a long way. My feet are no longer as hypersensitive as they were the first year after my stroke. I couldn't bear anyone running into my feet accidentally. Sixteen months post-stroke, I treat myself to a massage once a month. It feels good when the masseuse stimulates my feet or when I rub them.

I never believe the occupational therapists who work with me at Emory's Brain Health Center when they say, "If I don't bend your index finger and thumb now, they'll never bend." Dr. Milton used to give me a thumbs-up. I'd respond with a thumbs-up that looked like I was pointing a gun at him. Funny! The occupational therapists suggest that I might have arthritis or something else. Nope. *They don't know what the heck they're talking about,* I think. *I know my body.* As with my feet, I must remind myself that my right hand has greatly improved. When I make a thumbs-up now, it looks more like a thumbs-up, even though my thumb won't yet extend its full range, and my index finger won't tuck under completely; at least it's not sticking straight out. As with writing, I remind myself, *I've been here before, stuck.* The writing is a mess, despite all the time and effort I've devoted to it. But I know from experience that eventually the writing takes shape, because I persevere. My efforts and prayers pay off when I commit to the long game.

## Ambidexterity?

My left hand has assumed the slack of my right hand. I'm now somewhat ambidextrous. Neuroscientists describe brain plasticity as the ability of the brain to recover. Positive plasticity is when one brain area takes over the function of the other. Without thought, I grasp a glass of water with my left hand as comfortably as I would have done with my right pre-stroke. I clip the toenails on my right foot with my left hand. Most of the time, I intentionally use my right hand to retrain and strengthen it. I can hold a full glass of water in my right hand. But I cannot grab a practically full thirty-two–fluid-ounce bottle of Dawn liquid detergent without dropping it. I can stir a hot pot of greens with my right hand but must be careful because the hot steam will burn the tip of my index finger before I feel the heat.

Part 4: Home and Nineteen Months Later

## Blood Pressure

The doctors never provided an answer to my question, "What caused my blood pressure to spike so high?" That silence haunts me. How will I know how to prevent my blood pressure from spiking again? I don't want to be on blood pressure medication my entire life. But I likely will. One of my nurses at ERH tells me that her sister's blood pressure inexplicably spiked out of control when she was about my age and "postmenopausal." Actually, a woman is never postmenopausal; the menstrual period never returns, normally. The nurse says that her sister consulted with numerous doctors before finding one that provided an acceptable answer: menopause! Menopause can cause a woman's blood pressure to rise and remain elevated. I think both stress and the effects of menopause raised my blood pressure. But I'm uncertain.

My blood pressure stayed on the low side most of my life. At times in my life, I drank dandelion root tea and swallowed dandelion root capsules to raise my low blood pressure because I was near anemia. Stress can raise your blood pressure. Stress can kill you. Was I stressed out? Yes, I was, in retrospect. As already stated, the videos of police brutality and murder by police officer of Black and brown bodies stressed me out. I watched MSNBC's coverage of events, day and night. Between April 2022 and May 2023, a year before my stroke, I watched as Black men, children, and women were murdered by police. Rob Adams, Jayland Walker, Patrick Lyoya, Herman Whitfield, Jaylen Randle, Donovan Lewis, Eric Holmes, Joshua Wright, Tyre Nichols, Darryl Williams, Timothy Johnson, Irvo Otieno, James Lanier, Dexter Wade, and so many others. Black Americans were asphyxiated or shot and left to die in the streets by callous, often racist police officers. In 2022, police killed 1,266 people. In 2023, the number rose to 1,351. Black people are three times more likely than white Americans to be killed by police.[2]

## Sleep

I still require a lot of sleep. More precisely, I need a healthy dose of sleep. I've never slept so much in my life as I have during my recovery from stroke, not since I was a baby. I need nine hours, which is healthy for any human being

---

2. According to Mapping Police Violence, the numbers are even higher for Native Hawaiians and Pacific Islanders.

under normal circumstances. And some days, depending on how much I do in a day, I need a nap. When I nap, I may wake two to three hours later. I've come to accept that this is my new normal. Perhaps, if I had practiced sleeping nine hours pre-stroke, I'd have decreased my risk of stroke.

## Runny Nose

My nose runs whenever I eat—a full meal, a small sandwich, a piece of fruit, or even a stick of gum. Dang! It runs wherever I am. At home or in a restaurant. When eating in a restaurant, I grab all the napkins I can get. They pile up in dirty napkin wads like weeklong dirty laundry because the flow from my nose is constant once I start eating. It is as if my body is constantly cleansing and has yet to figure out that mealtime is a very inconvenient time to do so. I try to remember to carry enough tissues in my purse to catch the flow. I don't always remember. It is an embarrassing side effect of the stroke. If I'm eating with someone, I feel the need to explain, "My nose runs whenever I eat. It's a side effect of the stroke." They mostly say, "Don't apologize." Fortunately, I don't eat out too often. It's not healthy.

## Brain Fog

I feel in some regards that my thinking is sharper as I heal, but I also experience more moments of brain fog than before my stroke. I notice that the brain fog moments increase if I fail to get enough sleep.

## EMTs, Ambulance, and Medical Bills

I have great health insurance at CTS. However, we would all greatly benefit from quality, equitable, and affordable universal health care. There are always hospital bills due to deductibles, needing to use providers outside of one's network, and disputes between insurance companies and providers. The two Black male EMTs arrived at my home first in the wee hours of May 24, 2023 to assess my situation. Their assessment led them to call for an ambulance, which was driven by a white male and a Black male EMT; the white man could have been an EMT too. I'm not sure. The Black EMT who assessed me a second time in the ambulance gave me a baby aspirin, which I vomited up, documented my health and personal information, and shared it with the driver. That day, I was assessed by three Black EMTs, which is unusual, I'd imagine, outside of the Atlanta area. Only 6.6 percent of paramedics (or EMTs) are Black; 4.5 percent are Asian and even less are native Americans or indigenous Indians.

The name of the ambulance service is American Medical Response (AMR). My insurance company claimed I owe AMR no additional monies because of a prior agreement between the insurance company and AMR. AMR continued sending me letters demanding that I pay them a little more than $2,300, despite the paperwork I had sent them from my insurance company. More than a year post-stroke, I continued to be harassed. Turns out my insurer made an error and has now paid AMR. The high cost of ambulance service and such harassment might deter some people from using an ambulance. And privatized ambulance services might also motivate some ambulance businesses from serving poor people, if the primary goal is profit. In Georgia, on Thursday, December 5, 2024, Amanda Sylvester, a fifteen-year-old African American girl, collapsed at a volleyball practice and died from cardiac arrest after an ambulance failed to show up. A Dream Chasers Volleyball Club member, Amanda fell ill while warming up at the Tracy Wyatt recreation complex in an Atlanta suburb of College Park. EMTs arrived within minutes and evaluated the teen, but an ambulance that was called never came.

# 53

# Epilogue

I DO NOT SHARE the belief that God is the cause of sickness or evil. I don't believe that God is sitting around waiting for something horrible to happen to us so that God might teach us a lesson or make us stronger. Human beings create poverty, racism, sexism, heterosexism, ageism, environmental injustice, climate change, and other evils that negatively impact individuals and communities. I don't share the belief that trials and tribulations are the best ways that God can instill in human beings wisdom, strength of character, or resilience, even if testimonies of some biblical characters support such a conclusion. Testimonies are subjective, as Michael Newheart and I have written in *We are All Witnesses*; they reflect the experience and understandings of the testifier. Testimonies are not necessarily objective or universal; they don't reflect all experience. There's no way that the voices of the few communities or individuals codified in our Bibles (Protestant, Catholic, or Orthodox) represent all of human experience or interactions with God or God's Spirit. The author of the Letter of James testifies that "When being tested [Greek: *peiradzomenos*], let no one claim, 'I am being tested by God.' For God is untestable [Greek: *apeirastos*] by bad things, and God herself tests no one" (1:13; my translation). The community to which he or she is writing is going through some tribulations or hardships and experiencing internal class and cultural conflict that require more than the rhetoric of faith; "works" or actions are necessary. In a recent conversation with theologian, art historian, peer mentor, and friend Dr. Sheila Winborne, she argued that perhaps "God is often trying to teach us wisdom and not an easy certainty. It's about maturity. . . . we are on a wisdom journey," within our particular contexts. James is one of her favorite biblical texts.

I have committed to do all that I can do to be as healthy as I can be, to do the necessary work. Some hours, days, and weeks are and will be more difficult than others. I would like to think and was taught to believe that once I've done all I can do—which is relative, contextual, arguable, and subjective—God will do the rest. But so many people die after having done all they can do. To make life fit our theologies, we shift our thinking to blame the victim by saying, "They must not have done all they could have done." Can anybody really meet that standard when faced with fascism, racism, sexism, xenophobia, capitalistic greed, and poverty? Too many helpless children—in Congo, Gaza, US, Cameroon, Israel, in other war zones—who suffer and die at the end of having done all they can do to survive and live also share that hope in God. But God doesn't show up. We, as Black women and men, shared that hope during the 2024 presidential election, but most of us were devastated. Perhaps we can count on what Ta-Nehisi Coates advises: "You are called to struggle [against oppression, evil, sickness], not because it assures you victory but because it assures you an honorable sane life."[1]

All our theologies are hope. God, in all her inscrutability, transcendence, and unpredictableness, is our hope and beyond our hope. Our hope does not buy us privileges that other human beings don't have access to. Our hope does not guarantee our survival. Our socioeconomic and geographical context or sociocultural capital may assure us access to privileges that make the things we hope and pray for more accessible and achievable. All our theologies are fragile and contextual. God remains unpredictable. Everything does not always turn out alright! Does our theology teach us to become accustomed to being alright with what's not alright? Where does that leave us in terms of political involvement and social justice activism? Or with a faith *plus* works/action theology? I cannot help but conjure or invoke the God-language I was taught at home and indoctrinated with in church. It is my language of faith origins. We are encouraged to adjust our thinking or circumstances to accommodate the commodifying theology we were taught could be bought with our tithes, church attendance, modest dress, pure speech, and so forth. If God is unpredictable, the impact of human indifference, greed, and hatred is very predictable. Who escapes?

---

1. Coates, *Between the World and Me*, 97.

## Epilogue

I did not write everything I wanted to say, but I hope what I have written is helpful to my readers. I can't remember everything. Bits and pieces come back to me, in their own time. Time and timing has a say in every act of writing. I decided to write my memoir while on study leave from my institution (late August 2024 through January 27, 2025). Writing this memoir was not part of the study leave plan I submitted to Dean Yoder (and to the Trustee Board). I have other necessary things to write before my study leave ends, when I resume my other commitments of teaching and meetings. Some things must be left unsaid. Some things cannot be written because my recovery continues. I'm still living my story, for which I'm grateful. I have committed to do all that I can do to remain healthy. That's all I can do. The rest is out of my hands.

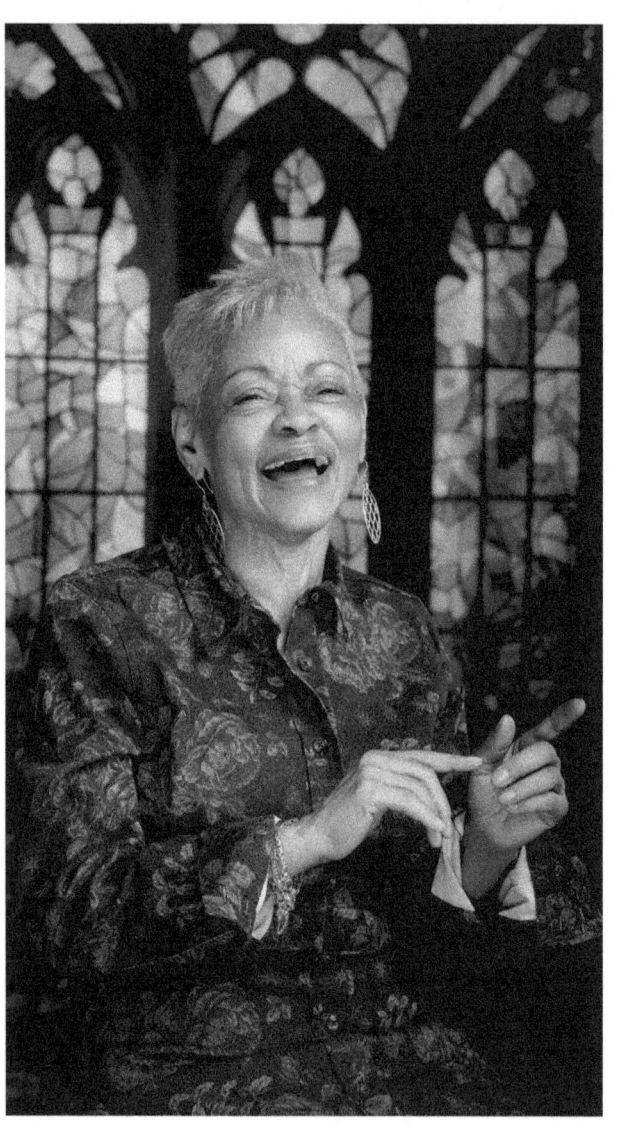

# Appendix

# Reproductive Justice, Medical Apartheid, and the Gospel of Matthew[1]

IN HIS FEBRUARY 6, 2024, Brite Divinity School McFadin Lecture, Corey D. B. Walker described abolitionist Christianity as "disruptive, not fixated on being included in empire building or 'burning house' . . . [It is disruptive] of the imperial logic . . . [and] injects new meaning into the world and in a new humanity what it means to be human in the world." Walker asked, "What if it comes from Black folk, ordinary Black folk, [Black women], brown folk, queer folk?" Walker further argued that "abolitionist Christianity is inconvenient and disruptive of the normal." Walker quoted Karl Barth's 1911 declaration: "Jesus is the movement for social justice and the movement for social justice is Jesus in the present."[2]

We learn about Jesus's life and ministry, of course, from the Gospels; they are not autobiographical. We access the Jesus of the Gospels through the interpretative lens of others and through the translations/interpretations of dominant interpreters. And often our readings of the Bible, including the Gospels, are not critical readings of depictions of Jesus or God.

---

1. The following is my first presentation after my stroke. It is the keynote address presented at the 2024 annual conference of the Society for the Study of Black Religion (SSBR) held in Nashville, Tennessee, on March 21, 2024.

2. Brite Divinity School, "McFadin Lecture with Corey D. B. Walker."

## Appendix

Dominant interpreters have taught us that the ancient biblical text is more sacred than the lives of Black and Brown folk and of women who stand in front of the biblical text—living, breathing readers. Dominant interpreters have also taught us that the ancient world behind the text is more significant than this racialized, misogynistic, and queerphobic/transphobic world and the communities therein, where Black and Brown people must negotiate life, living, and death. Abolitionist humanity must read the Bible and the Jesus or God depicted therein critically but not exegetically. Reading exegetically, or exegesis, implies and often demands a binarized hermeneutical perspective that requires or pretends an objective reading out of a text as opposed to a cultural, contextual reading into or with the Bible (so-called eisegesis). We cannot afford to ignore but must privilege, unapologetically, our own contexts in hermeneutical or interpretative tasks. Exegesis demands that we treat the world in front of the text where we live only marginally and lastly, if at all. It asks that we replace our own ability and right to read critically and against the grain with the commentary of dominant white interpreters.

So, as a biblical scholar, I start with the world in front of the biblical text where Black folks, Black women, and other humans live; our lives are sacred. I read issues of injustice against humanity, especially Black women, men, and children, in conversation with and as the lens or framework for critical dialogical readings. Here I focus on two passages from Matthew's Gospel: first, the story of Herod's massacre of the innocent babies, and second, the narrative of the Canaanite woman. I read these texts through the lens of reproductive justice/injustice and medical apartheid, respectively. I am personally familiar with the health care system or medical apartheid because my mother was in constant need of health care and, more recently, as a patient myself after suffering three mild strokes. The first, it seems, occurred when I attended the SSBR in DC last year, and the final stroke happened in the wee hours of the morning on May 24, 2023. I experienced both excellent and horrifying health care.

The children of Black women (especially of poor Black women) are subjected to a lower quality of life than their white counterparts through systems, structures, laws, policies, and practices that devalue, refuse to protect, and criminalize Black life while tolerating and normalizing violence against Black women and the children they birth. We know that pro-life activists love Black women's embryos and fetuses but hate the Black flesh that they encounter in this world. According to the Centers for Disease

Control and Prevention (CDC), "In 2021, the maternal mortality rate for Black women was 69.9 deaths per 100,000 live births, 2.6 times the rate for White women (26.6). Rates for Black women were significantly higher than rates for White and Hispanic women. The increases from 2020 to 2021 for all were significant."[3] White supremacy wasted no time transforming Black enslavement into the mass criminalization and incarceration of Black people. As Toni Morrison states, the "slave body is the Black body."[4] The school-to-prison pipeline or the disproportionate incarceration of Black men and women is enslavement by another name.[5] White supremacist nationalism will do all in its power to keep Black mothers and their born children from possessing and exercising their citizenship rights with the full protection of the law and from having access to equal and living wages, affordable housing and unobstructed property ownership, quality health care, free excellent education, and so on. But to maintain the status quo of white supremacy dominance, Black babies must continue to be born into an underclass that whiteness constantly dominates at the expense of Black life and flourishing.

In Harriet Washington's *Medical Apartheid*, Washington recounts the painful, dehumanizing history of gynecological experimentation on enslaved Black women's bodies by J. Marion Sims, the father of modern gynecology, for the benefit of white women's survival and health.[6] Some things do not change. Racism, sexism, classism, queerphobia, and transphobia are forms of violence that impact Black well-being and health. Donna Christian-Christensen, MD, former chair of the Congressional Black Caucus Health Braintrust, stated that "health disparities are the civil rights issue of the 21st century."[7] Rachel weeps and cannot be consoled.

The recent US Supreme Court decision in *Dobbs v. Jackson Women's Health Organization* overturned *Roe v. Wade* (1973) and with it almost fifty years of legal precedence. Poor Black women, who experience the highest percentages of rape on the basis of race/ethnicity, will be forced to carry all pregnancies to term, despite the systemic diminishment of Black women's quality of life.[8] The Justices argue that Black children can be put into the al-

---

3. Hoyert, "Maternal Mortality Rates."
4. Morrison, *Source of Self-Regard*, 77.
5. See, for example, Alexander, *New Jim Crow*; Ritchie, *Arrested Justice*.
6. Washington, *Medical Apartheid*.
7. Quoted in Washington, *Medical Apartheid*, 3.
8. Thompson et al., "Race, Ethnicity, Substance Use, and Unwanted Sexual

ready overburdened and troubled foster care system or adopted out. Black children disproportionately age out of the foster care system without being adopted. Poor Black women experience difficulty locating affordable livable housing for themselves and their children. In his *Evicted: Poverty and Profit in the American City*, Matthew Desmond argues that while Black men are being incarcerated in large numbers, Black women (and their children) are disproportionately being put out onto the streets.[9]

In Matthew 1, Mary gives birth to a baby boy who is named Emmanuel, which means "God is with us." Throughout the Hebrew Bible, God reminds humans that God is with them; God works with humanity. In Matthew 2, God is with the baby Jesus and his family through other human beings. Wise men from the East have followed the star they saw in the eastern sky, and they eventually arrive in Jerusalem after Jesus's birth. They are seeking the geographical location of the baby whom they believe has been born and is destined to be the king of the Jews. The star has taken them so far and no farther; they must now seek human intervention to complete their quest. So, they humbly ask the townsfolk folks for assistance to find the location where the child has been born. The wise men could be Jewish, gentile, or Godfearers. Regardless, they propose to worship the royal child as only men of means can: with gold and expensive oils. Divine power functions in the collective work of humans across ethnicity, race, religion, gender, socioeconomic status, and sexuality.

Word about the nature of the wise men's inquiry reaches King Herod the Great, Rome's puppet king of Judea. Herod and all of Jerusalem are troubled by what they have heard. Herod is disturbed because of the potential threat this infant poses to his position and legacy, and the people are perhaps troubled because they know Herod's reputation for cruelty and hypocrisy. Herod summons Jewish high priests and scribes who, after consulting the writings of the prophets, inform Herod that the child would be born in Bethlehem of Judea. Herod resolves to murder Jewish babies and infants to keep one child from surviving. When empire or white nationalism is unsure which children of a particular race will challenge the status quo and raise a people up from the bottom, it targets them all.

Herod secretly summons the wise men who respectfully listen to him and agree that, when they find the child, they will return to Herod with the location so that he too can worship the child (2:16). Herod uses the same

---

Intercourse."

9. Desmond, *Evicted*.

language of worship (*proskuneō*) as the wise men—it is the rhetoric of both empire and the colonized; it is the speech of humility and of abuse of power. Herod intends to murder children. Men of power in patriarchal societies can do great harm to women and their children when motivated by fear of loss, fear of being replaced, or fear of becoming both marginalized and colonized like the masses they oppress.

The wise men believe in dreams; their ancestors taught them that dreams mean something. They choose to embody the epistemologies of their ancestors *and* worship of God. As mentioned earlier, the wise men could be Jewish; they could be Egyptian Jews who did not view the study of the stars as antithetical to worshipping God or God's Messiah. Or they could be gentile polytheistic patrons of Israel's God. The fear that drives Herod to murder children must have been heightened by the gold and other expensive gifts the wise men planned to gift to the would-be king of the Jews, the baby Jesus. A poor Messiah is less of a threat than one with access to wealth; he might be more difficult to find and kill. He has means to flee. The child can be born, but he must die, if not today then tomorrow, or inevitably. If Jesus had not been identified as king of the Jews, as God with us, would the men from the East have traveled so far with treasure chests of gold, frankincense, and myrrh for the child's mother? Women and their children without social status and royal lineage, who live in "blackened" or stigmatized flesh, are considered unworthy of financial support and health care aid, let alone worthy of expensive gifts. Former President Reagan called poor Black women "welfare queens," and a politics of disgust resulted in middle-class women across race abandoning poor Black women. Consequently, many poor Black women were denied assistance, including health care. Racism and classism are forms of violence.

Indeed, God appears to be with Mary and assures her that her child will enter the world with purpose, and the wise men's gifts are the means to give the child a decent start in life, despite the fact that Mary had no choice in the matter of conception or birth. When society refuses to make the world a place where all children can flourish but insists that all mothers who conceive, regardless of the circumstances, give birth against their wills, parents and their children are less likely to survive and thrive. Today, Black women (and women in general) are more likely to die during childbirth than from an abortion.[10]

---

10. Raymond and Grimes, "Comparative Safety of Legal Induced Abortion and Childbirth."

Many folks will champion childbirth and demonize abortion and the disposal of unused embryos, but they will support laws and policies that disenfranchise poor mothers and fathers. The children of poor parents are expected to be the mules of society on whose bodies wealth and empires are built. Under the *Dobbs v. Jackson* decision, states are empowered to criminalize abortion, regardless of the circumstances under which the girl is impregnated and despite any real threat to the mother's life. While majority Republican-led states moved quickly in the wake of *Dobbs v. Jackson* to categorically criminalize abortion, they—and other states—have done little to find the many Black women and girls who continue to disappear. Over 60,000 black girls go missing each year, and in 2020 that number was almost 100,000, but they received little, if any, national media coverage.[11] Black girls go missing and are disappeared, mistreated, and murdered; their files are closed and their stories remain untold. If Rachel doesn't weep, who will? The website *Our Black Girls* tells the stories of missing, murdered, and mistreated Black girls and women because they have been forgotten and their cases archived and unsolved. Black children are more likely to be riddled with sixty bullets by the police while running away for fear of their lives, but white children and men who commit violent crimes can be treated to McD's en route to jail.

Racism, classism, sexism, queerphobia, and transphobia are a threat to Black health. Some people think we live in a post-racial society, but if individuals and groups fail to do the lifelong anti-racism work or therapy necessary for anti-racism reform and transformation, racism will likely still live within and raise its ugly head in the destruction of Black and Brown peoples and society. An unconscious racism is as deadly as intentional, overt racism. In her *Just Medicine: A Cure For Racial Inequality in American Health Care*, Dayna Bowen Matthew writes: "An unconscious racist unintentionally operationalizes historically and socially reinforced negative perceptions, judgments and behavior toward those from disfavored racial or ethnic groups through their implicit biases . . . Unconscious racism due to implicit bias is hidden, tolerated, and even excused despite its destructiveness; while implicit bias is not overt racism or bigotry the injustice and inequality that flow from both conscious and unconscious racism are equally egregious."[12] Further, Matthew argues, "Studies show that these implicit biases, whether accurate or inaccurate, will powerfully inform how

---

11. Pruitt-Young, "Tens of Thousands of Black Women Vanish Each Year."
12. Matthew, *Just Medicine*, 54.

the physician behaves with this new patient from the very first moment that they meet ... The fact that this physician's assumptions and stereotypes—his implicit biases—are neither irrational nor consciously chosen, does not mean that the discrimination that arises from them will not be extremely harmful to his new patient's health."[13]

God did not intervene to save the children Herod murdered. What kind of God will do for his son what she/he/they will not do for the children of others? What kind of God cannot or will not destroy the murderer to save the children? Perhaps the author of Matthew (likely an elite owner of enslaved persons)[14] could not imagine a God who intervenes to save certain children from a murderous king. Herod could not imagine God saving the children of those relegated to lower-class status, the children who are not among the talented tenth. He couldn't imagine a God who turns Matthew's world right side up for the least among us.

The world needs people and organizations that perform individual and collective acts of social justice—feeding the hungry, visiting the imprisoned, clothing the naked. But we must also be about the business of destroying unjust systems, structures, and policies. The Gospel of Matthew thrives on enslavement, as the many slave parables demonstrate. But those systems must not be replicated, even or especially those inscribed in a sacred text.

While some humans like the three wise men are committed to saving the baby Messiah's life, no humans intervene for the other babies and children—two years old and under—whom Herod murders. The children are disposable. They are the children of lazy, hypersexual "welfare Queens" and prostitutes; the children themselves are potential thugs, rapists, Jezebels, and "super predators."[15]

The violence of poverty, racism, sexism, transphobia, and queerphobia are interconnected with life expectancy and quality of life and care. In his *The Locust Effect*, Gary Haugen argues that the masses of people living in poverty globally cannot escape poverty as long as they are subjected to ineffective policing, violence, and exploitation.

Black women, regardless of their social status, give birth to babies who enter a world hostile to Black people and unable to breathe due to police brutality and environmental injustice. George Floyd, Frank Tyson,

---

13. Matthew, *Just Medicine*, 49.
14. See Smith and Jayachitra, eds., *Teaching All Nations*.
15. Riley, "Hilary Clinton Apologizes for 'Superpredators' Remark."

## Appendix

Breonna Taylor, Sandra Bland, Sonya Massey, and too many other Black people should still be alive! Poor women and their children have no place to go and no means to flee the violence. Joseph and Mary's baby, Jesus, is ultimately saved through fugitivity; the family is able to flee. Poor Black women and other poor women cannot afford to relocate to receive better health care or access abortion care.

The wise men who travel to welcome Jesus's birth are warned in dreams to avoid Herod; they flee, returning home by another route. Only men receive dreams in Matthew's story. The mothers of the murdered children receive no warning and thus cannot escape Herod's death sentence. After Herod dies, an angel tells Joseph to take his wife and child and return to Israel (2:19). But when Joseph hears that Herod the Great's son, Archelaus, succeeded him as ruler over Judea, Joseph is afraid to return to Judea (2:22a). Consequently, in another dream, Joseph is instructed to immigrate to Nazareth (2:22b). Interestingly, the last warning comes as the result of Joseph's fear. Joseph's fear doesn't keep God from helping the couple.

At critical junctures in the narrative (the search for the baby Jesus, the birth, the state-sanctioned murder of children, fugitivity, and immigration), the narrator inserts the words "this was to fulfill," or this was done so that the words of the prophet Jeremiah or other prophets might be fulfilled. Those words encourage readers to uncritically accept the depiction of God as most concerned with the existential reality of his Son and to justify the murder of the innocent babies and toddlers because the one child who matters in the story is saved and because it was foretold in the Scriptures, according to the narrator. But this thinking encourages readers to read from a position of privilege where many of us do not live and to feel no need to comfort Rachel in the only way she can be consoled—through justice. Sébastien Doane argues that "Rachel did not have a chance to mourn the death of her children, [which] causes us to lean toward a metaphorical interpretation of Rachel's weeping."[16] As long as Rachel's children enter into the world in stigmatized flesh and suffer and die because of their stigmatized flesh, the cycle continues without justice; Rachel cannot be consoled. Dána-Ain Davis argues that

> Black women are *at risk*, and they are *a risk*. When something (or someone) is considered to be a risk, a state of unease takes over . . . Risk can contribute to states of anxiety, to which the response is various forms of governmentality . . . Simply *being* Black

---

16. Doane, "Rachel Weeping," 5–6.

indexes distrust and precipitates profiling and assignment into risk categories based on nonthreatening behaviors. Labeling is a dangerous endeavor ... How is it, one might wonder, that women who have given birth fit into categories of risk? Or [how] is it that racialized bodies are in constant need of surveillance regardless of circumstances? Again, it is hard to know, but this is the kind of uncertainty that plagues many Black people in the United States.[17]

Doane asks, "Why does God ignore and abandon the other families of Bethlehem?"[18] His answer is that God *does not* spare his Son from the fate of the other children: "He died in the same way as the children of Bethlehem: murdered at the hands of the politico-religious authorities of Jerusalem. Jesus identifies with the suffering of the people"; he escapes but returns and is subjected to "the same violence, but he subverts it."[19] Thus, according to Doane, Jesus's crucifixion unexpectedly disrupts the cyclical violence, and the dead children are symbolically raised with Jesus.[20] Conversely, I propose that Jesus had the chance to live his life to maturity—to live into his potential and to live to reach adulthood; the other children did not. Our grave sites are rife with unfulfilled potential. Their lives and futures mattered too. God does not intervene for Rachel's children through angels, wise men, or parents able to flee the violence. Just as God sent his Son into the world in human flesh to accomplish for humans what God could not do as God, human beings must be agents of wholeness for other human beings, for one another. We must be human abolitionists.

Perhaps God cannot or will not do for humans what God created humans to do for one another. As in the Yahwist version of the story of creation (Gen 3), God did not find God's self to be a suitable helper for the human being God created; it had to be another human being.

The murders Herod orders are executed by human beings and no other human beings intervene. Doane asks a necessary question: "How can we attribute divine guilt when we ourselves are doing nothing to prevent injustice and death?"[21] Throughout the story, human beings intercede on behalf of the baby Jesus but not for the other babies and children whom Herod murders. Injustice flourishes when human beings cannot be

17. Davis, *Reproductive Justice*, 107.
18. Doane, "Rachel Weeping," 12.
19. Doane, "Rachel Weeping," 13.
20. Doane, "Rachel Weeping," 13.
21. Doane, "Rachel Weeping," 15.

inconvenienced to prevent it, or fear inhibits our actions. Evil seems propelled by fear, but fear paralyzes good people. Sometimes our faulty theologies inhibit us from being human abolitionists: God is in control; thus, we do nothing except pray, and we wait on God when, all the while, God is waiting on us. Or we say, "It was the victim's time to die." But as long as we do nothing to disrupt injustice, the Rachels of the world weep and cannot be consoled.

Perhaps we will tire of mourning over injustice and do our part as individuals and collectively. If Rachel doesn't mourn, who will? As long as unjust systems, structures, policies, and practices flourish, Rachel cannot be consoled. Injustice that is allowed to flourish will eventually impact everyone; it will sooner or later find its way into our back and front yards. In the meantime, Rachel refuses to be consoled.

## Naming the Injustice and Calling Her Name

The nameless mother in Matthew 15:21–28, identified as a Canaanite woman, has a daughter whose body is tortured by a demon. This mother is another human being negotiating life in stigmatized "blackened" flesh, flesh that is subjected to disdain and bias. She approaches a man named Jesus, who has a reputation for healing, and asks him to restore her daughter to health.

In the first century CE, healing and healers were not rare. In his *Zealot: The Life and Times of Jesus of Nazareth*, Reza Aslan argues that Jesus was known as one of those healers who healed people for free.[22] Certainly, this is the impression we get in the Gospels, that Jesus healed many within the orbit of his travels for free. And some people *not* within Jesus's path heard that he was healing folks free of charge, and they sought him out, as did the Canaanite woman. She likely heard stories of Jesus's miracles and perhaps saw the evidence. Surely, he would not hesitate to rid her daughter of the so-called demon destroying her body and slowly taking her life.

The Canaanite woman is identified broadly by her ethnicity or provenance; she is not an Israelite—she and her daughter are foreigners in relation to Jesus. While two Canaanite women, Tamar and Rahab, are mentioned in Matthew's genealogy, they are included because they birthed significant male children whose fathers were Israelites and who are supposedly related to David and to Jesus. The Canaanite woman is treated as

22. Aslan, *Zealot*.

## Reproductive Justice, Medical Apartheid, and the Gospel of Matthew

an outsider, not an insider, despite the mention of Tamar and Rahab in the genealogy. Inclusion often does not include parity, nor does it guarantee nice treatment, especially in racialized, patriarchal, queerphobic societies.

This Canaanite mother approaches and addresses the man Jesus with a desperately loud cry; she too is weeping. The NRSV and other translations characterize her as shouting loudly, as if she is angry and annoying. It matters who translates. Her plea is concise, direct, and to the point. "Show me mercy. Master, King David's son, my daughter is tormented by a demon." We have no idea how old the woman or her daughter are; we know the situation is dire, even life-threatening. This Canaanite mother has come to the only urgent care, ER, ICU, hospital to which she has access. Unfortunately, the first response to her plea for mercy is dead silence from Jesus: He does not answer her at all, the text says. We don't know how long the silence lasts, but silence in a life-and-death situation is an inhospitable, to say the least, and painful response; in fact, desperate need met with silence is emotional and psychological violence and may cause further physical harm depending on the circumstances. The response of the church to the many missing trafficked children in Atlanta and nationwide is largely silence. Former President Trump's initial silence about the COVID virus caused many unnecessary deaths, which disproportionately impacted Black people. Silence is not a compassionate response in this situation. I know that we often want to give Jesus a pass, but I wish we could let him be human, as human as the folks to whom he is related in his genealogy, especially King David.

A little over nine months ago, I went to the urgent care on Ponce in Atlanta. When they took my blood pressure, it was far too high: 176/110. The young Black nurse seemed alarmed but said nothing. The South Asian doctor whom I saw said he didn't know what to say, even after I told him my feet were numb and painful. He didn't listen well to my story; I told him I had vomited once several weeks ago after returning from a trip to DC—he sent me away with a prescription for nausea medication. I threw it away. I couldn't tell if he was that inexperienced or didn't care. Either way, the response was harmful. On May 24, 2023, I entered the ER in excruciating pain, having suffered a third and worse minor stroke. While I waited, the stroke continue to damage my body.

Silence in an emergency situation can mean the difference between life and death. Some folks preach that Jesus was testing this woman. It is cruel to test a person during a life-threatening situation.

The silence is broken by the cruel words that Jesus's disciple speaks to him in the woman's presence: Send her away! The last woman I shared a hospital room with was a Kenyan American who had worked in hospice care but suffered a stroke while having brain surgery. She understandably did not want to move when the therapist would come early in the morning to get her out of the bed—she had paralysis, I did not. But I didn't want to get up the first couple of days. A few of the nursing staff, and most of them were Black women, were talking outside our room and I could hear them say that she was not ready to be here; she needed to be sent home. I was mortified that this conversation was happening in our hearing.

Although the Canaanite woman is anonymous, for our purposes I am naming her *Eimi-Anthropé* (I am a human being). *Eimi-Anthropé*'s humanity or human need are not sufficient for the disciples to advocate for her, to encourage Jesus to help her. Instead of advocating for the woman, they turn on her. Dayna Matthew states that the "racial biases held by health care workers other than physicians have been ignored: nurses, physician extenders, technicians, and even medical staff workers such as receptions, administrators, and insurers are also likely unconscious contributors to health disparities."[23]

Jesus breaks his silence with words that are exclusive, dismissive, and lack compassion: "I was only sent to the lost sheep of the house of Israel." Jesus breaks his silence to deny *Eimi-Anthropé*'s plea because of her ethnicity; she is not a wayward Israelite! It is because of what she is *not* and not because of what *Eimi-Anthropé* is that she has yet to receive the response from Jesus that she needs and deserves. When I was a master's student in the Black studies program at The Ohio State University in the mid-1980s, I was researching cancer incidence and mortality rates for Black people and whites in the Ohio counties with the largest Black populations. The incidence rates in almost every form of cancer was lower for Black people, but the mortality rate was higher, apparently due in part to their difficulties accessing the best cancer treatment facilities and care. (Apparently, we now have both higher incidence *and* higher mortality rates.) In the process of my research, I located a news article in which a white doctor stated that many of his peers did not believe Black people deserved the best care even when they had good insurance. While, before Trump, it became socially unacceptable to be overtly racist, some are still trying to take us backwards.

---

23. Matthew, *Just Medicine*, 37.

As Dayna Matthew writes in *Just Medicine*, racism, whether intentional or unintentional, is harmful. Further, patients as well as doctors show up in the hospital or doctor's office with their own experiences and expectations. The doctor's conduct will be filtered through experiences and expectations.[24] In turn, "The doctor, having stored her own stereotypes as well, may 'read' the patient's behavior through the lens of her unconsciously held stereotypes."[25]

*Eimi-Anthropé* cannot, does not, give up. She cannot give up, despite the silence, disrespect, biases, and discouragement to which Jesus and his disciples subject her. Perhaps she came knowing the hoops through which she might have to jump.

When I was ill, I resisted going to the ER until my pain was unbearable. At times I felt I was improving; perhaps it was a virus. Also, I'd been in the ER too many times with my mother while she was living. Often the silent waiting was long and the treatment by staff disappointing, to say the least. I thought that I was likely to die in an ER. But when the pain became intolerable, I called 911 and was taken to the ER where I waited for hours shivering in the cold air conditioning for tests and an almost empty space at 3:00 AM. It wasn't until I attempted to sign the ER admittance papers that I discovered I could not write my name. The stroke was taking its toll as I waited. The MRI would reveal I had had three minor strokes, the third and worst that early morning on May 24. Although I felt I would die in the ER, I endured to get the help I needed. *Eimi-Anthropé* had no choice but to endure the insults in the hope of getting the help she needed for her daughter. So, *Eimi-Anthropé* knelt on the ground and repeatedly begged, "Master, help me!"

Not all human beings can be moved by human misery, suffering, and need. But I think Jesus is moved with compassion when *Eimi-Anthropé* confronts his ethnic bias and disparity. Matthew writes that, "when differences [in care] are related solely to race and ethnicity, they become 'disparities' and are unjustifiable."[26] Jesus, with the help of *Eimi-Anthropé*, will work through what he had been taught about the superiority or election of Israel. Jesus's response to her continual pleading is an insulting metaphorical saying that re-emphasizes Israel's priority over other peoples: "It is not fair to take the children's bread and cast it to the dogs." *Eimi-Anthropé*

---

24. Matthew, *Just Medicine*, 52.
25. Matthew, *Just Medicine*, 53.
26. Matthew, *Just Medicine*, 30.

challenges Jesus's words while also using his words against him and in her favor: "Indeed, Master, for even the small dogs eat the crumbs that fall from the table of their master." A compassionate master allows the pets to eat while the children eat. *Eimi-Anthropé* envisions a more compassionate master or patriarch of the household who ensures that all living creatures in the home eat; they don't have to wait. No one goes without what they need to live.

God created all and desires all living things to have what they need to survive and thrive. Human need or suffering should be sufficient reason to receive the compassion of God and should be enough for us to demonstrate compassion toward our fellow humans and other living creatures. The God who has worked and does work through Jesus also works in other humans who believe in a compassionate God—the God who has no name—who shows no favoritism.

Ultimately, Jesus replies to *Eimi-Anthropé*: "O Woman, Great is your faith; let it be done to you as you wish." Jesus does not say that he himself healed *Eimi-Anthropé*'s daughter; rather, the healing comes from *Eimi-Anthropé*'s resolve and resilience. It is the omnipotent narrator who tells the reader that *Eimi-Anthropé*'s daughter was healed that very hour. *Eimi-Anthropé* endured silence or indifference to her desperate plea for help, the disciple's hurtful words urging Jesus to dismiss her, ethnic bias, and the trauma of her and her people being called a bitch. But *Eimi-Anthropé* never gave up on her daughter or Jesus; her daughter deserves to be healed because she too is a human being who needs healing!

According to Dayna Matthew, research shows that "implicit bias can be *intentionally* reversed. Therefore, the preponderance of malleability evidence warrants a complete reconceptualization of when and how providers could and should be held accountable to intervene and thwart the discriminatory impact of unintentional racial and ethnic discrimination."[27] But, Matthew states, "Implementing the transformation to an equitable health care model must be borne of the conviction that continued avoidance of the evidence that implicit bias causes disparities, and that disparities ruin lives, will be unethical at best, unjust indeed, and patently unforgivable."[28]

In this story of the Canaanite mother, we find the Greek words *megalé sou hé pistis* (her great faith). In fact, this is the only place we find this phrase in the New Testament. On the one hand, *Eimi-Anthropé* is commended. On

---

27. Matthew, *Just Medicine*, 170.
28. Matthew, *Just Medicine*, 172.

the other hand, why must she demonstrate great faith for her daughter to be healed? And what is great faith? How is it measured? By the amount of trauma and dehumanizing bias one is willing to endure for health care? In Matthew 17:14–20, Jesus tells his disciples that, if they had the faith the size of a mustard seed, they themselves could have healed the boy possessed of a demon; they could move mountains. Why should *Eimi-Anthropé* demonstrate great faith before her daughter is healed? *Eimi-Anthropé*'s daughter's human need should be sufficient for a loving God to facilitate her healing. This story reminds me of the respectability politics to which too many marginalized people are subjected.

When it comes to human need, God is no respecter of persons. When I was in the rehab hospital, I shared a room with one other stroke victim. Our room had no shower, just a sink and toilet; we either had to learn to wash ourselves from a small plastic tub or were given a bed bath by a nurse. I didn't know that some hospital rooms in the newer section of the building had showers. I don't know for whom those other rooms were reserved or if they were first come first served. One day, a part-time nurse named Georgia arrived around 6:00 AM, and she came into my room to ask if I wanted a shower. In shock I asked, "How are you going to do that?" She said, "Don't worry about it, do you want one?" I said, "Yes." Evidently, it was Georgia's habit and hers alone to treat three patients with various degrees of disability to a hot shower whenever she was there. This was my lucky day. I felt renewed after the shower. Georgia was my angel. God is like Georgia, or Georgia is like God. God is interested in meeting human need and alleviating human suffering. May we find a way to do our part as individuals and as a collective.

# Bibliography

Adichie, Chimamanda Ngozi. "The Danger of a Single Story." YouTube, October 8, 2009, 19:16. TED Talk. https://youtu.be/D9Ihs241zeg.

Alcindor, Yamiche, et al. "With a History of Abuse in American Medicine, Black Patients Struggle for Equal Access." PBS, February 24, 2021. https://www.pbs.org/newshour/show/with-a-history-of-abuse-in-american-medicine-black-patients-struggle-for-equal-access.

Alexander, Michelle. *The New Jim Crow: Incarceration in an Age of Color Blindness*. New York: New Press, 2012.

American Heart Association. "Facts, Causes and Risks of Stroke." Last reviewed February 16, 2024. https://www.goredforwomen.org/en/about-heart-disease-in-women/facts/facts-causes-risks-and-prevention-of-stroke.

———. "Let's Talk About Risk Factors of Stroke." 2023. https://www.stroke.org/en/help-and-support/resource-library/lets-talk-about-stroke/risk-factors.

American Heart Association News. "Is It Fatigue—or a Stroke? Women Shouldn't Ignore These Warning Signs." May 31, 2019. https://www.heart.org/en/news/2019/05/31/is-it-fatigue-or-a-stroke-wome-shouldnt-ignore-these-warnig-signs.

Aslan, Reza. *Zealot: The Life and Times of Jesus of Nazareth*. New York: Random House, 2013.

Bolte Taylor, Jill. *My Stroke of Insight: A Brain Scientist's Personal Journey*. London: Yellow Kite, 2022.

Bridges, Khiara. "Implicit Bias and Racial Disparities in Health Care." In "The State of Health Care in the United States." Edited by Jane Perkins. Special issue of *Human Rights Magazine*. https://www.americanbar.org/groups/crsj/publications/human_rights_magazine_home/the-state-of-healthcare-in-the-united-states/racial-disparities-in-health-care/.

Brite Divinity School. "McFadin Lecture with Corey D. B. Walker, February 6, 2024." YouTube, February 7, 2024, 61:2. https://www.youtube.com/watch?v=kEdBnyoYNMg&ab_channel=BriteDivinitySchool.

Coates, Ta-Nehisi. *Between the World and Me*. New York: Spiegel & Grau, 2015.

Comaford, Christine. "Are You Getting Enough Hugs?" *Forbes*, August 22, 2020. https://www.forbes.com/sites/christinecomaford/2020/08/22/are-you-getting-enough-hugs/.

Cornish, Stephanie. "Study: Black Patients Treated With Less Compassion Than Whites." *AFRO: The Black Media Authority*, January 29, 2016. https://afro.com/study-black-patients-treated-with-less-compassion-than-whites/.

# Bibliography

Davis, Dána-Ain. *Reproductive Justice: Racism, Pregnancy, and Premature Birth*. New York: New York University Press, 2019.

Desmond, Matthew. *Evicted: Poverty and Profit in the American City*. New York: Crown, 2016.

———. *Poverty by America*. New York: Crown, 2023.

Doane, Sébastien. "Rachel Weeping: Intertextuality as a Means of Transforming the Readers' Worldview." *Journal of the Bible and Its Reception* 4 (2017) 1–20. https://doi.org/10.1515/jbr-2017-2000.

Elders, Jocelyn. Speech at the One Hundred Forty-Second Annual Meeting of the American Public Health Association. YouTube, November 18, 2014, 8:5. https://www.youtube.com/watch?v=bzORS85svqE.

Foxx, Jamie, and Hamish Hamilton. *Jamie Foxx: What Had Happened Was . . . Written by Jamie Foxx*. Directed by Hamish Hamilton. Netflix, 2024.

Haugen, Gary. *The Locust Effect: Why the End of Poverty Requires the End of Violence*. Oxford: Oxford University Press, 2014.

Hong, Cathy Park. *Minor Feelings: An Asian American Reckoning*. New York: One World, 2020.

Hoyert, Donna L. "Maternal Mortality Rates in the United States, 2021." National Center for Health Statistics. https://www.cdc.gov/nchs/data/hestat/maternal-mortality/2021/maternal-mortality-rates-2021.htm.

Johnson, Josh. "The Almighty Payout: LA Archdiocese Settles for $880 Million." YouTube, October 23, 2024, 26:9. https://www.youtube.com/watch?v=M-7Mp4JLDVs.

Kendrick, Anna, dir. *Woman of the Hour*. Netflix, 2023.

Mapping Police Violence. https://mappingpoliceviolence.org/.

Matthew, Dayna Bowen. *Just Medicine: A Cure for Racial Inequality in American Health Care*. New York: New York University Press, 2015.

Morrison, Toni. *The Source of Self-Regard*. New York: Vintage, 2020.

NeuroLaunch Editorial Team. "Walking Brain: The Surprising Benefits of Movement for Cognitive Function." September 30, 2024. https://neurolaunch.com/walking-brain/.

Office of Minority Health. "Stroke and African Americans." US Department of Health and Human Services. September 22, 2023. https://minorityhealth.hhs.gov/stroke-and-african-americans.

Orminski, Emily. "Sleep Is a Cyclical Inequity for Those in Poverty." National Community Reinvestment Coalition. August 5, 2021. https://ncrc.org/sleep-is-a-cyclical-inequity-for-those-in-poverty/.

Pruitt-Young, Sharon. "Tens Of Thousands Of Black Women Vanish Each Year. This Website Tells Their Stories." NPR, September 24, 2021. https://www.npr.org/2021/09/24/1040048967/missing-black-women-girls-left-out-media-ignored.

Quist, Donald Edem. *To Those Bounded*. Austin, TX: AWST, 2021.

Raymond, Elizabeth G., and David A. Grimes. "The Comparative Safety of Legal Induced Abortion and Childbirth in the United States." *Obstetrics and Gynecology* 119 (2012) 2015–19. https://doi.org/10.1097/aog.0b013e31823fe923.

Riley, Katie. "Hilary Clinton Apologizes for 'Superpredators' Remark." *Time*, February 25, 2016. https://time.com/4238230/hilary-clinton-black-lives-matter-superpredator/.

Ritchie, Beth. *Arrested Justice: Black Women, Violence, and America's Prison Nation*. New York: New York University Press, 2012.

## Bibliography

Sabin, Janice A. "How We Fail Black Patients in Pain." Association of American Medical Colleges (AAMC). January 6, 2020. https//www.aamc.org/news/how-we-fail-black-patients-pain.

Simmons, Avery. "Why We Need More Black Physical Therapists." PracticePromotions. net. https://practicepromotions.net/black-physical-therapists/.

Smith, Mitzi J., host. Beyond the Womanist Classroom podcast. Season 2, Episode 4, "Religion and Horror," featuring Dr. DeAnna M. Daniels. August 2, 2024. https://mitzijsmith.net/beyond-the-womanist-classroom-podcast/.

———. *Insights From African American Interpretation. Reading the Bible in the Twenty-first Century*. Minneapolis: Fortress, 2017.

Smith, Mitzi, and Jayachitra Lalitha, eds. *Teaching All Nations: Interrogating the Matthean Great Commission*. Minneapolis: Fortress, 2014.

Smith, Mitzi, and Michael W. Newheart. *We are All Witnesses: Toward Disruptive and Creative Biblical Interpretation*. Eugene, OR: Cascade, 2023.

Thompson, Nancy J., et al. "Race, Ethnicity, Substance Use, and Unwanted Sexual Intercourse Among Adolescent Females in the United States." *Western Journal of Emergency Medicine* 13 (2012) 283–88. https://doi.org/10.5811/westjem.2012.3.11774.

Walker, Alice. *In Search of Our Mothers' Gardens: Womanist Prose*. San Diego: Harcourt Brace, 1983.

Washington, Harriett A. *Medical Apartheid: The Dark History of Medical Experimentation on Black Americans from Colonial Times to the Present*. New York: Harlem Moon, 2006.

www.ingramcontent.com/pod-product-compliance
Lightning Source LLC
Chambersburg PA
CBHW032226080426
42735CB00008B/737